THE RENEWAL
OF
PERSONAL ENERGY

David E. Hunt

Introduction by Seymour B. Sarason

Monograph Series / 25

OISE Press / The Ontario Institute for Studies in Education

The Ontario Institute for Studies in Education has three prime functions: to conduct programs of graduate study in education, to undertake research in education, and to assist in the implementation of the findings of educational studies. The Institute is a college chartered by an Act of the Ontario Legislature in 1965. It is affiliated with the University of Toronto for graduate studies purposes.

The publications program of the Institute has been established to make available information and materials arising from studies in education, to foster the spirit of critical inquiry, and to provide a forum for the exchange of ideas about education. The opinions expressed should be viewed as those of the contributors.

Canadian Cataloguing in Publication Data

Hunt, David E., 1925-
  The renewal of personal energy

(Monograph series ; 25)
Includes bibliographical references and index.
ISBN 0-7744-0368-3

1. Self-perception. 2. Self-actualization
(Psychology). 3. Vitality. 4. Burn out (Psychology) —
Prevention. I. Title. II. Series: Monograph series
(Ontario Institute for Studies in Education) ; 25.

BF637.S4H8   1991   158¹.1   C91-095783-5

Typesetting: Sharon Richmond
Cover Design: Sheila Barnard
Editor: Frances Rooney

ISBN 0-7744-0368-3   Printed in Canada
1 2 3 4 5 AP 69 59 49 39 29

To Jan
with love and appreciation
for renewing my life

Contents

INTRODUCTION

One of the features of adult development is the way we find ourselves changing our perspectives about ourselves, our work, our family, and a lot else. The degree of change may be large or small, fast or slow, accepted or resisted. We like to believe that we change because of a rational process by which we have looked truth in the face and confronted the ineluctable: we had to change. It is my observation that those who have a most difficult time contemplating the need for change and facing up to its consequences are people who have been very successful. Rewarded for their success by whatever criteria appropriate to their work, they do not look kindly, when they look at all, at truly personal change. For example, if you are a researcher whose studies have brought you respect, recognition, and elevated status, it is understandable that you will resist listening to that small voice within that suggests that what you thought was the truth was otherwise. It is not a voice that says you got the facts wrong but rather that you put them into a wrong or too limiting a context of assumptions and values. And, as often happens, that small voice speaks up when you are no longer enamored with your work, when you sense you are or will be repeating yourself in your work, when you are puzzled by the fact that however you explain your feeling, you are explaining only a small aspect of the phenomenon — when these combine with the voice within, you have a problem. In that kind of situation, some retreat, many waffle, and a few have the courage to come to grips with the issues. It is not a personal-professional conflict that anyone can wholly avoid, surface appearances to the contrary notwithstanding.

In his previous book, *Beginning with Ourselves* (1987), David Hunt had the courage to describe in instructive detail the changes he has gone through in an illustrious research career. He has always been a person who could take distance from himself, that is, look at himself, his work, and his field. So, when in that book Hunt tells us that each of us has to start "in here" with ourselves, he was talking from experience and not theory. And we should begin with ourselves because that is what we know best. That does not mean, Hunt said, that all that we know about ourselves is valid by whatever criteria of validity are ordinarily invoked. What it does mean is that each of us possesses knowledge of ourselves, with which we have to *begin*. I underline "begin" to emphasize Hunt's point: it is the beginning of a process and by no means the whole process.

It is characteristic of David Hunt that he tells us right off in the present book that he underestimated the difficulty people would have beginning with themselves. It is also characteristic that he sought to understand why this is so, why it has to be so, and he began to develop means to facilitate the beginnings of the process. And, again typically, Hunt makes an important distinction between change and renewal. You can change without necessarily feeling a renewal of energy, a truly energetic embracing of an altered view of self and future. His phrase "renewal of personal energy" is kin to what we mean by "rejuvenation": to experience again that outlook and energy level we had as youngsters that drew us to the future.

We have to start with ourselves. It initiates a continuous process facilitated by *sharing*. So, again, we start with ourselves but we end up with others.

Hunt states that the problem of burnout among helping professionals is reaching crisis proportions. I agree. The reasons are many — historical, political, economical, organizational — but they all converge to deplete the personal energy of too many people. Although Hunt's work started in the arena of education, he was wise and knowledgeable enough to know that the phenomena he was getting at had enormous relevance, not only for teachers, but for nurses, day care workers, counselors, social workers, and he says, "those responsible for sustaining the energy level of others, that is, administrators." Hunt is not one of those panacea seekers or proclaimers. Quite the contrary. What we have in this book is a continuation of a search for ways of *Beginning with Ourselves* in order to experience *The Renewal of Personal Energy*. This book is about and for all of us.

Seymour B. Sarason
Yale University

PREFACE

Whether your experience of personal energy is high or low, bursting or draining, you are all familiar with the topic of my book. Yet despite the importance of personal energy, and its renewal, in our daily lives, it is surprising that the topic has received so little attention. In contrast, we hear a great deal about conserving and renewing physical energy resources such as gas and oil. I believe that conserving and replenishing personal energy deserves the same attention we have devoted to natural energy resources.

Therefore, I offer you an invitation to connect with your own energy and to try out some of my ideas for renewal. Because of the current crisis in professional burnout, I direct my invitation first to those in the helping professions: teachers, nurses, counselors, consultants, day-care workers, social workers, and trainers, but I hope my ideas and approaches will also be valuable to theorists, researchers, and non-professionals; personal energy knows no bounds. I do not promise a quick fix for one-minute renewal, but rather a way to start connecting with your own energy and its potential for rejuvenation.

Like my earlier book, *Beginning with Ourselves* (Hunt, 1987), this book is based on experience — my own and others' — not on formal theory and experimental research. Therefore, I invite you to take it on experiential grounds and try it for yourself. Does it fit with your own experience of personal energy? Does it provide ways to enhance your self-knowledge? Do the ideas and approaches help you connect with your energy? Does it provide a meaningful basis for your own journey of renewal?

You may find in reading and trying my ideas that they are similar to earlier theories and approaches. I do not discuss these similarities, but colleagues have mentioned that my notions are similar to a wide variety of other ideas such as humanistic psychology, New Age ideas, hermeneutics, feminist theory, and psychosynthesis. I leave it to you to draw the parallels as you will. What is more important is that you accept my invitation to sense the personal meaning and value of my ideas for yourself. One colleague compared my approach to that of Roberto Assogiolo's *Psychosynthesis* (1965) saying, "Your approach is like psychosynthesis without roots." I agree that I do not provide the roots of a formal theory; rather I offer seeds for each of you to nurture into your own theory.

Also like *Beginning with Ourselves*, this book owes a great deal to my student/ colleagues in my graduate classes in the Focus on Teaching program in the Department of Applied Psychology at the Ontario Institute for Studies in Education. Student/colleagues in my Learning Styles class (now re-titled Practitioners' Experienced Knowledge) provided almost all of the examples in Chapters Three, Four, and Five, and equally important, helped me grasp the true meaning of "Learning is teaching, teaching is learning." I am equally indebted to student/colleagues in my doctoral seminars who contributed to the chapter Research as Renewal. I hope this chapter will not only broaden the meaning of renewal, but also will serve as a foundation for future researchers, especially experienced practitioners who have become researchers temporarily in conducting their doctoral thesis research.

My experience in working with these talented, experienced practitioners has been the keystone to developing my ideas, and I am indeed fortunate to have had this opportunity. Perhaps only at the Ontario Institute for Studies in Education might I have had this good fortune, and I am grateful for this as well as the continuing support that OISE has provided for my renewal. I have also been greatly supported and stimulated by my colleagues in our informal Educational Development Discussion Group, whose contribution goes considerably beyond their specific help as described in Chapter Two. The "Thursday Group" has opened my eyes to sharing as co-creation.

Several individual colleagues made valuable suggestions on earlier drafts, and for this I am grateful to Mary Beattie, Ardra Cole, Laura Ford, Anna-Liisa Leino, Jarkko Leino, and Harry Schroder. I feel a special sense of appreciation to Seymour Sarason for his exemplification, through his writing and his actions, of what I have discovered to be my basic values as well as his continuous encouragement through all my work on this book.

Thanks to Leslie Ireland and Julia Pine for their fine work in typing this manuscript and to Jennifer Wiberg for compiling the index. If it is "reader-friendly," much of the credit goes to copy editor Heather Berkeley, whose talent for unobtrusively bringing my voice out more clearly is much appreciated.

D.E.H.
September, 1991

CHAPTER ONE

Beginning With Ourselves: The Key to Energy Renewal

"Energy = internal or inherent power; capacity for action"
Webster's Dictionary

Our personal energy is a vital factor in our daily lives at work and at home. We know the feeling of being full of energy, whatever our personal description for this high energy experience may be: enthusiasm, buoyancy, exuberance, or bursting. By contrast, we know the feeling of being drained of energy, whether we think of it as emptiness, boredom, or flatness. We are also aware of changes in our energy level as it increases or decreases. These fluctuations not only produce different feelings, they also influence how well we get along at work and at home. When we are full of energy at work, we are more effective, more likely to try new approaches and learn new ideas. When our energy is at a low ebb, we find it difficult to keep at the job, let alone try new approaches and ideas. How well we get along with those close to us at home is also strongly influenced by our energy level.

Stop for a moment to reflect on your present level of energy. Connect with your present feelings and consider these questions: How would you describe your present energy level? How has it changed recently? Why has it changed? Chances are you are better able to recall how your energy has changed — whether it has increased or decreased — than to recall why these changes occurred, or how to replenish your energy when you feel drained. Your reflections ought to give you first-hand experience of the importance of the renewal of personal energy.

Each of us experiences our sense of energy in a distinctly personal way, yet there are a few general characteristics of personal energy: (1) it influences our feelings and our mood; (2) it influences our outlook and our perceptions; (3) it influences our actions; (4) it fluctuates over time; and (5) it remains at least partly mysterious.

Given its importance in our lives, it is surprising that the topic of renewing personal energy has received so little attention. We are told a great deal, perhaps more than we want to know, about professional burnout (e.g., Farber, 1991). We also hear about conserving physical energy resources, such as gas and oil, but little about the conservation and replenishment of human energy resources. One exception is Ingall's (1975) book *Human Energy* in which he conceptualizes the nature of human energy and provides some theoretical models for considering its sustenance and replenishment.

Renewal has received attention from several authors in the past decade, notably Gardner (1982), Waterman (1987), and Bolin and Falk (1987). Although Gardner's book is entitled *Self-Renewal*, it is actually concerned with societal renewal, while Waterman's *The Renewal Factor* is concerned with organizational renewal. Societal and organizational renewal provides the context within which personal renewal occurs, and I discuss this interplay in Chapter Six.

The work of Gardner and Waterman is similar to mine in our common concern with distinguishing renewal from change. For example, Gardner draws the following distinction:

> Renewal is not just innovation and change. It is also the promise of bringing the results of change in line with our purposes. (1982, p.7)

Waterman makes a similar distinction:

> Renewal, after all, is about builders. Many people can introduce change for change's sake and call it renewal. This is illusory. A builder, on the other hand, leads an organization to renewal that outlives the presence of any single individual, and revitalizes even as it changes. (1987, pp. 23-24)

In distinguishing renewal from change, I emphasize that renewal begins "*in here*," within ourselves, initiating a *continuous* process which is facilitated through *sharing* (as elaborated in Chapter Four). I define renewal as the process of connecting with personal energy, of releasing it, and transforming it into action.

Renewal usually refers to the professional development of experienced practitioners, but I will extend its range to other persons and other activities. Although most of my examples come from experienced practitioners in the helping professions, the concept of renewal applies equally to beginning professionals and to pre-service professional education. It also applies to non-professionals and to all of us when we are not at work; personal energy knows no boundaries. Renewal also applies to many areas beyond professional development: program initiation, team building, training, retraining, and even research (Chapter Seven). Personal energy is usually ignored in discussing these activities, so I will show how its inclusion sheds light on past failures and how to avoid them in the future.

I portray renewal through two major themes: (1) the relation between our personal images and our personal energy and (2) the Spirit of Renewal framework. In the first theme, I show how our personal images are connected to our central values, and therefore allow access to personal energy which is released and transformed into action through sharing. Using our personal images represents one specific means of renewal. In the second theme, I explore the Spirit of Renewal at a more general level, as portrayed in a framework of values, images, and qualities. This framework is applied to various activities (e.g., pre-service professional education and the renewing organization).

In this chapter, I begin by summarizing the major points in *Beginning with Ourselves* (Hunt, 1987) since they are the foundation for my major themes. Next, I describe *experienced knowledge*, the central feature of inner life which makes renewal possible.

Beginning With Ourselves: An Inside-Out Approach

If I have learned anything since writing *Beginning with Ourselves* (Hunt, 1987), it is that accepting the invitation in my title is much more difficult than it seems. I don't know how many times I have said to an individual, to one of my classes, or to a workshop, "The title means just what it says — begin with yourself, do not begin out there." To begin with ourselves is to stop and reflect, to enter into our inner life, to connect with what we feel and believe, and to set an inner foundation for continuing our life's journey. We not only go inside at the beginning of these reflections, but we retain a firm connection with our inner lives as we leave the world of reflection to enter the world of action.

My invitation to take an *Inside-out approach*, to begin with our inner feelings and beliefs, contrasts with an *Outside-in* approach where we focus on other people, outside experts, media, or external conditions (Hunt, 1987). In making the distinction between Inside-out and Outside-in, I am aware that I am making an oversimplification which raises many questions: Doesn't what is inside our hearts and heads originally come from *outside*? How do we go from inside to outside to enrich our inner lives? I propose the exaggerated dichotomy because I find an enormous tendency in many people to be cut off from themselves, to be unaware of their most precious feelings and central beliefs, and accordingly to lose confidence and feel dispirited. That is why the first step in the renewal process is to begin with ourselves, to stop and reflect, to connect with our inner wisdom.

Why this seemingly simple invitation should be so difficult and arouse such resistance is a very complex question which if dealt with completely would require another book. The psychological as well as the historical and contemporary cultural factors which have led so many of us away from our own selves, sometimes actively fleeing self-knowledge, are varied and subtle. However, I must deal partly with potential resistance to the approach, as I tried to do earlier (Hunt, 1987), because otherwise you will either stop reading or miss my experiential argument.

The most valued source of direction for my ideas comes from my graduate course originally entitled "Learning Styles and Teaching Approaches" and now called "Practitioners' Experienced Knowledge." This is essentially an extended workshop for experienced practitioners in human services — teachers, consultants, counselors, social workers, nurses, industrial trainers, and so on. It is not only that these student/colleagues continue to enhance my learning and provide almost all of my examples, but they also allow me to learn a great deal about resistance and how it can be overcome.

Resistance to connecting with our inner experience, to seeking self-knowledge, takes many forms: skepticism of anything that is not rational, recalling earlier negative experiences with attempts at self-understanding, dismissing Inside-out as touchy-feely activities for the tender minded, feeling inadequate about one's inner knowledge and imagination, and so on. Whatever your resistance may be, I must deal with it in this book so that I can persuade you to accept my invitation to try to renew yourself. If you do not try out my ideas, they will not receive a fair hearing, for I make my case for personal energy renewal on a personal, experiential basis. I believe that personal energy can be understood or communicated only through direct experience. Therefore, I frequently refer throughout the book to ways of overcoming your resistance.

For those of you who like to know the rationale of any invitation before accepting, I summarize the major points in favor of going Inside-out.

Why Inside–Out?

Every person is a psychologist

This stinger (a short, stinging statement that usually describes a basic assumption; it might be called a motto, maxim or one-liner) is based on George Kelly's (1955) belief that each of us in our daily lives develops implicit theories about human affairs, even though we are often unaware of doing so. We form miniature psychological theories about ourselves and others — how to communicate, how to influence, and how to foster development, as well as how we see ourselves. Like Freud, Rogers, and Skinner, we are theorists, too, having formulated beliefs based on our experience even though we have probably not validated our theories. Based on this assumption, Kelly proposed that the best way to understand others was to discover their underlying beliefs about human affairs, or what he called their "personal constructs" (1955). He offered this suggestion to clinicians who were attempting to understand their clients, but it is no less appropriate for each of us in non-clinical settings.

Another of my favorite Kelly stingers is his belief that as we grow older we develop "hardening of the categories." I have found that one antidote to this condition is to reverse stingers to gain a new perspective. Let's try this and see what happens.

Every psychologist is a person

I expressed this stinger originally in a paper, "Theorists are persons, too" (Hunt, 1978), which did not make a big hit with my psychologist colleagues. Psychologists strongly resist my suggestion because it strikes at the heart of their claim to expertise. Like all experts in human affairs, psychologists base their expertise on their role as detached scientific observers who function impersonally as they build their "knowledge base." No wonder they resist my suggestion so strongly! Having perpetrated my share of impersonal theories in my day, I sometimes try to surprise my audience by observing that one of the benefits of being a psychological theorist is the opportunity to elevate your personal beliefs to the level of scientific truth. In stating his *Reflexivity Principle*, George Kelly (1955) noted that psychology is a unique discipline in that the theorist is both a perpetrator of theory about and a participant in the phenomenon in question, human affairs.

Denying their personhood helps support the experts' illusion that words count more than actions. Imagine, for example, that you are attending a large lecture by an educational expert on how to personalize learning. Intuitively, you are aware that the lecture itself is an example of a learning situation, and that the lecturer's actions completely contradict what the lecturer is saying. Yet relying on logic and rationality, experts tend to ignore their own actions while exhorting others to change theirs. Since experts are not "mere persons," like the non-experts in their audience, they need not consider what their actions communicate. No wonder theory typically fails to influence practice!

Experts maintain their impersonal role to retain their authority, power, and control over non-experts. To accept that they are persons, too, would topple them from their detached positions of authority and erode their professional basis for power and control. Realizing that my proposal was threatening, I extended it to redefine the role of psychologists and to assure them that by accepting their personhood they would not be out of job. In their new role, psychologists would aim:

1. to foster self-understanding in themselves and others,
2. to facilitate communication and share understandings, and
3. to apply shared understanding to specific concerns. (Hunt, 1980, p. 293)

I think these activities would keep all psychologists busy, but so far my proposal has fared no better than my reversed stinger.

There is nothing so practical as a good theory

This stinger from Kurt Lewin (1952) describes the conventional view of how theory influences practice. Borrowed from the physical sciences, the sequence involves: (1) deriving a logical theory, (2) validating it with controlled research, (3) developing programs based on the validated theories, and (4) applying the programs in practice. Lewin's stinger was my motto for several years (Hunt, 1987, pp. 17-28) as I tried to apply my validated theories of personality development and learning style to classroom practice. However, I found that this sequence described neither how I was able to collaborate with the teachers nor the results of our work.

I discovered that when teachers adopted my notion of matching their approach to student learning styles, it was not due to the logic of the theories or to their research validation. What counted were my actions in communicating with them, specifically, whether I adapted to their styles in our communication as I hoped they would adapt to the styles of their students. In retrospect, I realized that an "Exemplification Principle," expressed as "Actions speak louder than words," was at work. Of course, I did not always follow my own principle (because, among other reasons, I was not then aware of it), but when I did communicate my ideas by my own example, I realized that they were more likely to be considered by the teachers with whom I was working. Teachers who adopted my notion of matching ideas also did so because my suggestions were very close to their own beliefs and practice. Taking account of teachers' present beliefs and actions was at least as important as my exemplifying my ideas.

Obvious as it seems, the role of teachers' current beliefs and practices is almost always ignored when new educational approaches are being recommended. We know that effective communication requires our taking account of the listener's viewpoint and "flexing" to their perspective, yet we forget its importance in practice-theory relations. All of us act according to our beliefs, and teachers are no exception. Therefore, their beliefs, or experienced knowledge, must be considered and respected in attempts to initiate new approaches. Once I realized the vital importance of teachers' implicit theories, I wrote "Teachers are psychologists, too" (Hunt, 1976), and I was on my way to an Inside-out approach to thinking about practice-theory relations even though I did not then realize it. I did realize, however, that it was time to reverse Lewin's stinger, not just to relieve my impending rigidity, but to proclaim a motto that would more truly define and direct my work.

There is nothing so theoretical as good practice

This stinger captures my belief that applied psychology, or any other applied discipline, must begin with practice. Put another way, unless theory comes directly from practice, it will not influence practice (Hunt, 1987, Chapter 7). With the zeal of the newly converted, I set out to spread the word about my new-found ideas. With

Richard DeCharms, who was visiting OISE at the time, I wrote a paper by this title, but it was summarily rejected. Next, I proposed to the journal Theory into Practice that they reverse their title to Practice into Theory (Hunt, 1980, p. 293). The title remains unchanged, of course, but much to my surprise, my paper was later selected as one of the five best on teacher development in the journal's 25 years of publication. I was left to ponder whether (1) they had not read the article or (2) the award was based on humor. It was about this time that I decided I must be on the right track because I was meeting increasingly stronger resistance.

I was not alone in reversing my motto as I discovered when I read Donald Schon's proposal for improving theory-practice relations by "turning the problem upside-down" (Schon, 1987, pp. 14-15). While my proposal came from my experience, Schon's argument was based on a critique of technical rationality, the logical foundation for the conventional theory-to-practice sequence. My argument was also supported by a RAND study review on the necessary conditions for successful educational innovation (Berman & McLaughlin, 1978). This monumental eight-volume review documented the necessity for the primacy of practice — beginning with teachers and local planning — for successful educational innovation. I was delighted to discover both an analytical basis from Schon and an empirical basis from RAND to support my view.

With such strong evidence for beginning with practice, why is the resistance so strong? It can only be that the idea of theory into practice is more than a motto or journal title, that it is embedded in more fundamental beliefs about the nature of thought and its influence on our actions. We seem to need to believe that the mind controls the body.[1] Reframing the mind—>body relation to body—>mind or to body<—>mind profoundly disturbs the prevalent world view that logic and rationality come first in human affairs. When it is seen as part of the mind-body problem, resistance to reversing this stinger becomes more understandable. Nonetheless, there are a few signs that we are shifting to the primacy of practice, the most noteworthy being the influence of Schon's suggestions on professional educational programs in general and teacher education specifically (Grimmet & Erickson, 1988).

Turning the theory-practice problem upside down so that we begin with practice highlights the central importance of practitioners' experienced knowledge, a notion which I summarize in the next sections.

Experienced Knowledge

Experienced knowledge is defined as our accumulated understanding of human affairs which resides in our hearts, heads, and actions. It guides our actions even

---

1. I am indebted to Richard de Charms for pointing at this relation.

though we are often unaware of this influence. Experienced knowledge is similar to earlier concepts such as personal constructs (Kelly, 1955), common-sense theories (Heider, 1958), and personal or tacit knowledge (Polanyi, 1962) as well as to more recent concepts such as professional knowledge (Schon, 1983; 1987), experiential knowledge (Brackman, 1976), personal theories (Fox, 1983), and personal practical knowledge (Connelly & Clandinin, 1988). The following assumptions show how experienced knowledge is distinguished from these other concepts.

On the nature of experienced knowledge

1. Every person's experienced knowledge is unique. To paraphrase Kluckhohn and Murray (1948), every person's experienced knowledge is (a) like *all* other persons' knowledge in some ways, (b) like *some* other persons' knowledge in some ways, and (c) like *no* other person's knowledge in some ways.
2. Personal knowledge is usually unexpressed so that its importance is often unacknowledged.
3. It is not necessarily true and valid; like formal theories, our experienced knowledge needs to be evaluated by observing our knowledge-in-use. However, it must be brought out in a non-judgmental atmosphere before applying critical judgment to observe its validity.

On domains of experienced knowledge

4. Experienced knowledge may refer primarily to our professional domain of work or to the *personal* domain which includes our activities at home. Knowledge in these areas is closely related since it comes from the same person ("personal" in another sense), but it is useful to distinguish the two domains.
5. Experienced knowledge in a professional domain is rooted in our experience of that domain before entering training. For example, the experience of teachers-to-be in the domain of education is the foundation for their experienced knowledge as they begin their pre-service professional education.

On bringing out experienced knowledge

6. Experienced knowledge is usually identified by recalling a past *experience* from which that *knowledge* may be brought out.
7. It is best identified by recalling *positive* experiences since these contain our resources and sources of energy. For example, a "positive" professional experience is one which we recall with positive feelings, even though parts of

it may have been quite challenging, and even negative. Once identified through positive experiences, experienced knowledge can be directed to address negative experiences or concerns.

8. Finally, each of us is responsible for discovering and defining our own experienced knowledge as well as determining how it will be shared and applied; it cannot be adequately defined by someone else, expert or not, and similarly, the decision to make such knowledge public and to share it belongs to those persons themselves, not to outsiders, experts or not.

Identifying Your Experienced Knowledge

We often say we learn from experience, yet we pay little attention to what we learn, to our experienced knowledge. Try the following exercise to get a first-hand sense of how we derive knowledge from our own experience. As indicated, experienced knowledge is not explicit so you may bring out knowledge you were not aware of earlier (i.e., your hidden resources).

The exercise follows the principles listed above so you begin by recalling a positive professional experience you can remember fairly clearly. Select an experience which made you feel good about yourself as a professional (the particular situation will depend on your role, of course, so it may involve teaching, counseling, administrating, or whatever your professional activity happens to be). If these do not apply to you, select any positive experience.

Find a sheet of paper, preferably unlined, and divide it into four sections by drawing three horizontal lines across the page so that there are four rectangles on the page. Number each space on the left-hand side form 1 to 4. Now you are ready to begin.

The first step is to try to remember the experience you have chosen as intensely as possible. Begin by recalling when it happened — the time of day, the day itself, the season of the year (don't write what you recall, do it in your head). Next, recall where the experience happened and reset the stage for it. Now that the stage is set, place yourself *in* the situation. Allow all the people who were originally there to become part of the scene. Make certain you are *in* the scene, not observing it. Now, before you re-experience the situation as it occurred, try to open all your senses to it — to the sights, sounds and smells, and especially to what you were feeling. The more vividly you can recall the experience, the more meaningful will be the knowledge which you bring out of it. Now, for a few moments, allow yourself to experience that experience as fully as possible. Don't write anything down, close your eyes, go inside, and recall your experience, focusing especially on your feelings in that moment. Take 30 or 40 seconds.

The second step is to come back from the experience and to consider the highlights. Jot these down in Box 2 on your sheet of paper. Don't be concerned with order or organization. You may want to write down feelings, what was said, parts of the scene, or whatever. Take about a minute to jot down a list of highlights.

In Box 2 you have summarized the main features of the experience, and now the third step is to put the parts together. So re-read what you have written in Box 2 and then in Box 3 answer the questions: Why did this experience work so well for me? What were the reasons for the success? What was the meaning of what happened? Can I explain it? Think about the experience for a few moments, then write down your understanding of it in Box 3. Take one or two minutes.

The fourth and final step is to reconsider your understanding of the experience, jotted down in Box 3, and then in Box 4 write out the implications for action. Re-read your understanding of why the experience worked and then write down a blueprint indicating the steps to take so that you would be likely to create another positive experience. Try to capture the "wisdom of action." Take one or two minutes to complete this final step.

You have gone through four steps in identifying your experienced knowledge, each step involving a different kind of mental activity. There is nothing written in the first box, yet in the first step of the exercise you were doing something. How would you describe what you were doing in a word or phrase? Participants often use words such as "recalling," "visualizing," or "experiencing." Write down the word which describes what you were doing on the right hand side of the paper. Do the same for the other three boxes. For Box 2, participants describe this with words such as "highlighting," "reflecting," or "listing." Descriptions of Box 3 involve words such as "analyzing," "interpreting," and "finding meaning." In Box 4, descriptions such as "planning," "taking action," or "implications" are used. Now let me reveal the lesson plan of this exercise. It is an experiential introduction to the experiential learning cycle proposed by David Kolb (1975; 1984) as shown in Figure 1.

Figure 1
Kolb's Experiential Learning Cycle

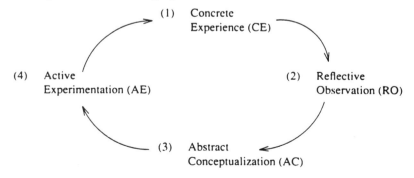

Source: adapted from Kolb, 1975. Used with permission.

Experienced Knowledge as Experiential Learning

The four-step sequence in the exercise is based on the four steps in the Kolb Cycle. Kolb believed that experiential learning could be considered in terms of four steps which in everyday affairs often meld together: (1) *Concrete experience* (CE) which refers to the original, direct sense of being in a situation; (2) *Reflective observation* (RO) which involves detaching ourselves from the experience to become an observer who reflects on the experience; (3) *Abstract conceptualization* (AC) which consists of putting the pieces together or theorizing about the experience; and (4) *Active experimentation* (AE) which involves initiating an action plan to experiment with the consequences or results of the action. The cycle continues with feedback on the action which leads to re-framing issues and continuing again through the cycle.

I am fond of playing variations on the Kolb Cycle (Hunt, 1987, pp. 150-156), and will continue to play variations on it throughout this book. For now, however, I want to use it as a source of identifying experienced knowledge from the exercise just completed. In the exercise you went through the four steps in the Kolb Cycle from Inside-out as shown in Table 1.

Table 1
Kolb Cycle from Outside-in and Inside-out

Steps in the Kolb Experiential Cycle (Outside-in)	Major Activity	Experiential Exercise (Inside-out)
1. Concrete Experience (CE)	Feeling	Experiencing Reliving
2. Reflective Observation (RO)	Perceiving	Highlighting Noting
3. Abstract Conceptualization (AC)	Thinking	Analyzing Making Sense
4. Active Experimentation (AE)	Acting	Planning Taking Acting

There are a few differences between the Kolb Cycle described above and the exercise I used to introduce you to it, because, first of all, the exercise involved recalling an experience rather than starting with direct experience and, second, it involved planning for action rather than actually taking action. Yet, the exercise gives a flavor of the Kolb Cycle, and depicts our learning through experience. Obviously, we do not go through all four steps in every situation and learning experience. Different situations call for emphasis on different parts of the cycle. For example, when we are engaged in our practice, we rarely have time for reflection and analysis. It is also true that we vary in terms of how well developed each of these modes has become for us. Some persons may be well developed in expressing their feelings, but not so well developed in their analytical capability.

This leads us to the first form of experienced knowledge we can extract from the exercise, our *self-perception*, or in this case, our awareness of our learning style. Think about your experience in the exercise, and try to answer the question, "Which one of the four steps was most difficult?" Difficulty may be indicated by not understanding the instructions, becoming distracted, or finding the other approaches interfering. Identifying which step was most difficult gives you an initial idea of your learning style according to the cycle. For example, if the first step, which involved remembering your feelings, was most difficult, you would be described as a "Southerner" (Hunt, 1987, pp. 150-156) because your well-developed modes in the cycle (Figure 1) are in the southern or lower portion. This orientation to the cycle leads to four patterns:

1. Underdeveloped CE   "Southerner"
   (or feelings)

2. Underdeveloped RO   "Westerner"
   (or perceiving)

3. Underdeveloped AC   "Northerner"
   (or thinking)

4. Underdeveloped AE   "Easterner"
   (action)

Which of these patterns best describes your learning style? Even though the exercise is brief, it provides a direct experience of the first form of experienced knowledge, *self-perception*, which I describe in the next section.

The experiential exercise also provides a beginning step for bringing out our *implicit theories*, the second form of experienced knowledge discussed here. Look back at your response in the third box, where you described why the experience you recalled was successful, and you will find the seed of your implicit theory about your professional life. For example, one participant wrote, "This happened because there was a feeling of trust between the students and myself which gave me a sense of confidence." Although brief, this account contains the foundation for an implicit theory of teaching practice. (Other examples will be given in the next section.)

The third form of experienced knowledge, *personal images* of our practice, is a topic I discuss in detail in Chapter Three. (You might begin to identify your personal images by following an imagery exercise in Appendix 1.) The remainder of this chapter discusses these three forms of experienced knowledge in order to show both how they vary and how they provide a reservoir of untapped resources for the renewal of your personal energy.

Forms of Experienced Knowledge

Self-perception

Self-perception refers to how we see ourselves now as well as how we think we were in the past and how we would like to be in the future. Often there is a relation between our self-perceptions and our implicit theories, especially the dimensions we think of as important in our implicit theories. For example, we may hold a personal dimension such as "talkative-silent" to be important, and it may serve as a basis of our self-perception. How would you see yourself on this dimension at present? And where would you like to be in the future? You might see yourself, for example, as having been talkative in the past and present, wishing to become less talkative and capable of silence in the future. In this case, a present self-perception sets the stage for future movement, a process I discuss in Chapter Eight.

Of the many varieties of self-perception, I have focused most extensively on identifying our own learning style and becoming aware of its importance. The following four examples illustrate the variety of learning styles as well as the four points on the Kolb Cycle.

1. Northerner: "I learn best when I can talk things through with colleagues to test my perspective. Many of my decisions are made emotionally and intuitively. I have difficulty conceptualizing unless I can identify the idea with specific examples."
2. Westerner: "My well-developed quality is listening and reflecting, and my underdeveloped mode is action. In order to act, I need an experience which draws out my thinking."
3. Southerner: "[I am an] analytical, logical thinker [and I'm] uncomfortable in unstructured situations. I need to know background theory, I'm not feeling-oriented, I need time to reflect before I act, and I'm somewhat uncomfortable in situations which require imagination and risk-taking."

4. Easterner: "I am a self-directed, action oriented learner who requires concrete application for practice, and a sense of comfort or security to progress. I don't take enough time to reflect or plan, though I feel things go better when I do."

What is the value of becoming aware of your learning style? The following quotation gives some indication:

> I'd never before sat down and thought about how I learned — through reflecting on my own actions. The process in this exercise reinforces the concept of the teacher as an experienced professional. The information I was seeking was there inside me all along, all I needed to do was channel and focus my energy to reflect on what the experience could tell me about the way I work best and learn best. I felt very refreshed and positive about this, as it reinforced and built confidence despite my initial feeling of insecurity about the subject matter.

Furthermore, if we accept the assumption that the major purpose of considering learning styles — our own and those of others — is to facilitate communication, then identifying our learning style may be a key to difficulties in communication. To emphasize this point, I use an "Opposite partners" exercise in which student/ colleagues who are opposite in their learning styles, for example, a Northerner paired with a Southerner, work together on a communication exercise. First, one partner selects a favorite hobby or sport which the partner also enjoys, and then communicates about the hobby using his or her well-developed mode. Northerners communicate about their hobbies through the "language of feeling," emphasizing what it feels like when they are involved in their hobby. Then their partner does the same except in the opposite "language." For instance, a recent pair happened to choose the same topic, gardening, but they communicated about it in very different ways, and by reference to very different gardens. The Northerner described her garden as a wild, unplanned panoply of color with no distinction between weeds and flowers. This garden gave her a sense of beauty and freedom. Her partner, a Southerner, described planning a meticulous garden in specific rows with the color patterns carefully plotted.

These initial descriptions are followed by each person's attempt to communicate using the "opposite language," and this is where the fun begins. Most participants find it very difficult to communicate in their underdeveloped modes, but nonetheless find it valuable to experiment with the wide variety of ways of learning and representing experience. Most important, they face the issue of how a mutually acceptable "language" is negotiated when partners are opposite.

Implicit theories

Implicit theories are the underlying beliefs we hold about the nature of human affairs, and they guide our actions in many areas, for example, how to communicate with another effectively, how to influence another, how to develop and grow, how to facilitate growth and development, and so on. In a series of exercises entitled, "How to Be Your Own Best Theorist," participants bring out their underlying beliefs in terms of their (1) perceptions or the dimensions of considering others and themselves, (2) intentions or their hopes and goals in working with others in their practice, and (3) their actions or the ways in which they work towards achieving their intentions. Perceptions, intentions, and actions are the inner representations of the Outside-in categories of student characteristics, learning goals, and teaching approaches which I have used earlier (Hunt, 1987).

Once these categories are identified, participants can begin working on their relationships to one another, for example, on how their perceptions influence their actions. If we see a student or client as "shy" (perception), what will be our action? One participant answered this as follows: "If I see students as shy, then I allow them to work alone so they will not feel uncomfortable." Bringing out the "If . . . , then . . ." of the relationship between perceptions and actions amounts to creating a matching model (Hunt, 1987), which is central to our implicit theories. Another participant might arrive at quite a different action from the same perception: "If I see students as shy, then I encourage them to come out of their shell by working with more outgoing students." These are not only different courses of action, but they flow from different implicit theories.

As mentioned earlier, the experiential exercise gives a beginning basis for identifying our implicit theories through considering the AC portion of the Kolb exercise. Following are four examples of implicit theories:

1. Self-confidence, self-awareness, and growth are important for successful learning. A supportive, positive class atmosphere, one of trust and responsible freedom, can be generated by students and teachers to enhance learning. A teacher is a guide on the side, not a sage on the stage.
2. Be specific! Be organized! Be practical! These are the messages for my instructors. Knowledge should be acquired for a specific reason. Do not waste time learning what you will never use. Discriminate and pursue the knowledge you can apply in your own personal journey.
3. Every individual has something worthwhile to contribute. We can learn from one another: everyone a learner, everyone a teacher. We learn best when we pool our resources. Learning occurs best in a safe, positive, nurturing environment.
4. Learning is the chocolate sauce of life. Learning is what makes life exciting and rich just as chocolate sauce adds sweetness, texture, and richness to an ice cream sundae. As a facilitator, I have the opportunity to sweeten many individuals' lives. I also have a tremendous opportunity to learn from my students by engaging in experiences with them to enrich my own life.

As the last example illustrates, implicit theories may be closely related to personal images (discussed next) since all forms of experienced knowledge emanate from a common source of central beliefs. As you read these examples, you probably agree with some and disagree with others, which raises the question, how do we check the validity of our implicit theories? When practitioners become their own best theorists, they assume the same responsibility as do formal theorists to evaluate their theories in practice. For example, your "experiment" might consist of taping a portion of your actions, as a sample of theory-in-use, in order to check on whether you are actually putting your theory into use and if so, whether it serves your intentions.

I have recently summarized an implicit theory of my own as a simple stinger to guide my actions: "Accentuate the positive." To show that it is more than a song title, I need to document its value and validity in my actions. When I consider my "stinger-in-use," I find that it almost always works. I have taped classroom or workshop transactions to check whether I am true to this motto and, if so, the effects that it produces. I found that by emphasizing positive qualities, participants are much more likely to take the risk of looking for inner wisdom. The value of this "stinger-in-use" has also been documented through anonymous evaluations and by the work of the student/colleagues as illustrated in their verbatim comments in Chapters Three, Four, and Five. "Accentuate the positive" began as a tentative motto, and has become a fundamental article of faith for me. Thank you, Johnny Mercer!

As I discuss in Chapter Eight, such stingers can be very valuable when they become stingers-in-use even though they initially appear to be superficial. If we use "Accentuate the positive" to gauge and direct our actions throughout the day, we will begin to understand its power and its role in the Spirit of Renewal described in Chapter Six.

Personal Images

Since personal images are central to one of my major themes (the relation of images to energy), I will devote several pages in Chapter Three to clarifying their meaning. Yet we can begin here by noting that personal images are inner representations of which we may only be vaguely aware. We may experience these personal representations as daydreams, fantasies, hopes, visions, or ideal conditions. As I discuss later, they are often non-verbal and they may be non-visual.

Since you may be unfamiliar with your own imagination, let's begin by imagining another person's image. This may not represent an image of your own, but it will get you started. Following is an image from a student/colleague, Sheila, who found that an image of a rushing stream was underlying her work as a consultant. As you read Sheila's description of her image, try to become the stream, enter into it, and make it your own. An outside image becomes a personal or inner image when you enter into it in your imagination.

> My image is that of a stream, bubbling, exploring, seeking new paths. As I pass there is growth — luxurious grass, trees, and fantastic flowers. However, I rarely look back. As I journey on, through ever-changing terrain, I meet and join with other streams. We mingle, swell, and grow stronger, but I am still me — individual in the whole. Sometimes we go our separate ways. I feel a sense of loss but I know it is important to follow one's purpose and direction. Now, joined with others, I value their presence. I can also see growth in the lands ahead.

This image has personal meaning to the colleague who brought it out, but it can be shared by each of us. Take a moment to become the stream. Feel the flow of the water. Enter into the image for a few moments. As you enter into the image, transform it to your own lights. As you make the stream your own, notice your feelings and your level of energy.

Summarizing Your Resources

Your experienced knowledge is an untapped resource waiting to be discovered and brought out. To summarize their inner wisdom in the form of self-perception, implicit theories, and personal images is very affirming for practitioners. It is a celebration of practitioners-as-experts, and such explicit acknowledgment of their inner resources stands in stark contrast to viewing them as deficient and needing first aid for their numerous weaknesses. When practitioners summarize their self-perception, implicit theories, and personal images on a single sheet as shown in Table 2, they create a resource which can be shared with others.

Table 2
Experienced Knowledge Summary

My resources

Self-Perception

I am a Southerner with a well-developed facility to analyze and conceptualize thoughts and ideas. As an analytical, logical thinker I desire to know the facts so that I can make informed, rational decisions and undertake responsible, reasonable actions. I am constantly organizing and integrating the events of my life.

My underdeveloped quality is my feeling orientation, my CE on Kolb's Cycle. When feelings surface they are immediately superseded by intellectualization and rationalization. Likewise a free imagination is called to order by a rational mind. Therefore I find imaging a very difficult process because my critic instantly assumes control and starts to analyze.

Implicit Theories

My implicit theories are summarized in the stinger "Respect and Expect!" To respect others means accepting them as they are with their developed and underdeveloped qualities, their individuality. To expect others to be their "best selves" means endeavoring to support and encourage each person to be, to do, and to give his or her best.

This respecting and expecting flourishes in a warm and caring environment where everyone is accepted, supported, and challenged to grow and where fairness, justice, consistency, and understanding are present.

Personal Images

My image is of myself holding a bouquet of multi-colored balloons attached to strings of various lengths. These balloons are unlike other balloons. They are not filled with air but rather with my developed and underdeveloped qualities. I experience the qualities of each balloon through the vibrating string that I hold in my hand. Some of the balloons are large (my developed qualities) and have long strings so they soar above the others. Other balloons are small (my underdeveloped qualities) with shorter strings so they tend to bob below the larger ones.

Other people around me are also holding balloons of varying sizes on varying lengths of string. It is awe inspiring to see the giftedness of the people around me! The fun part comes in sharing balloons because it gives my smaller balloons a boost and helps them soar a little higher. Or several of us may join forces with our large balloons, producing such creative energy that wonderful things happen! Maybe even the Dance of the Balloons!

Imagine being in a workshop with 25 others and receiving a summary of each participant's experienced knowledge. (See Appendix 2 for more examples of experienced knowledge summaries.) Reading this rich and varied material is one of the best ways I have discovered to affirm Practitioners-as-experts.

Bringing out experienced knowledge is the first of three steps involved in renewal. (I discuss the next two steps in Chapters Four and Five.) Here I want to convey an idea of the potential value of bringing out experienced knowledge in facilitating self-knowledge and setting the foundation for new actions.

Figure 2 shows the relationship between the three forms of experienced knowledge and our central beliefs and values.

Using this figure as a guide, participants are encouraged to reflect on their own summary sheets and to focus on the *similarities* and *differences* in the three forms of knowledge. For example, participants might note the similarities between their

Figure 2

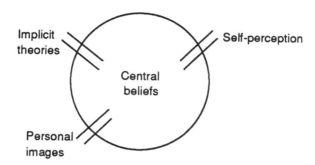

implicit theories and their personal images with an eye to consider how these relate to underlying values. What central beliefs do these theories and images represent? Participants may also use one form to stimulate another, for example, to ask what image is associated with a particular stinger or to try to express an image as a stinger.

Another way to further self-understanding is to ask, "Which of these three forms is most difficult for me?" Self-perceptions, implicit theories, and personal images are all ways to *access* our central beliefs and values, and some may be more accessible to us than others. This differential accessibility may be indicated by learning style. For example, participants who see themselves as Northerners, for whom feelings are very accessible, often report that imagery is more accessible to them than their implicit theories, while those who are Southerners, who tend to be analytical, find just the opposite. Discovering other access routes to your central beliefs is reassuring if you have found it difficult to connect with your personal imagery.

Once you have completed your reflections on your own knowledge summary, you may wish to peruse the summaries of others. Chapter Five deals primarily with how to use knowledge summaries for creative problem-solving in small group settings.

Plan of the Book

Chapter Two describes my discovery of the meaning of personal renewal, especially how it differs from planned change. I outline a renewal cycle which can be applied to individuals, to two-person transactions, and to small group transactions.

Chapter Three summarizes the nature and characteristics of *personal images* as distinct from *metaphors* and *symbols* on the one hand and from externally imposed images on the other. I provide evidence for the idea that identifying our personal images connects us with our personal energy.

Chapter Four introduces the idea of sharing as a form of co-creation which is essential to the releasing of personal energy. I also consider more generally the value of sharing in facilitating interpersonal relations.

Chapter Five describes the C-RE-A-T-E cycle, a small-group creative problem-solving approach based on the Kolb Cycle. I present specific instructions and illustrations of the cycle and document how its applications influence the release and transformation of energy.

Chapter Six develops a framework depicting the Spirit of Renewal in terms of values/beliefs, images, and qualities. The value of the framework is displayed by applying it to organizations, for example, the renewing organization and to pre-professional teacher education; teacher centers exemplify the Spirit of Renewal.

Chapter Seven discusses Research-as-renewal first in general through applying the Renewal framework and second with specific suggestions to researchers, especially practitioners who become researchers in conducting their doctoral theses.

Chapter Eight uses the image of a journey to discuss how we might renew our lives. Topics such as stress management, self-development, and avoiding external manipulation and control are considered within the image of a journey.

CHAPTER TWO

Discovering the Meaning of Renewal

"Renew: To make new again; to restore freshness or vigor"
Webster's Dictionary

In this chapter I describe why I selected renewal as the topic for this book. I follow my own advice, by beginning with myself as I try to show how I discovered the meaning of renewal during my sabbatical year in 1988/1989. Early in the year, I intended to write a book about change, so the major theme of this chapter is how renewal replaced change as my topic.

My ideas on renewal did not evolve through a series of "stepping stones" (Progoff, 1975), a process characterizing the development of some of my earlier ideas (Hunt, 1987, Chapter 2). It was more like working on a puzzle without having all of the pieces at the start. I had to identify the pieces of the puzzle, which turned out to be ideas such as *personal images, personal energy, creative problem-solving*, and *organizational support*. Then I had to study each piece and try to see how it would fit with the other pieces. All the pieces fell into place once I knew that my topic was renewal. When I returned from my sabbatical to be asked the usual question of what I had done during the year, I replied, "I discovered what I want to write about." Some people thought I was kidding, but I was quite serious. It was a year well spent.

Renewal is by no means a new concept, but it was a new idea for me, at least in the way I came to understand it. Yet when I reflect on what seem to be "new" ideas,

I am often intrigued to find that these "new" ideas appear, without my acknowledging their importance, much earlier in my thinking. For example, there was a 25-year lapse between my introduction by George Kelly in 1951 to the idea that "Every person is a psychologist" to my appreciating the idea's importance in education as reflected in the stinger "Teachers are psychologists, too" (Hunt, 1976). Reflecting on my more recent work, I first used the idea of renewal in a paper I presented in 1983, "Identifying your own learning style: a workshop in professional and personal renewal." At that time, I was using renewal in its traditional, more limited application to professional development rather than in its broader meaning discussed here. Still, the question lingers, What took me so long?

I began my sabbatical year with the vague idea of writing a sequel to *Beginning with Ourselves*, but I was uncertain of what I would write about. When I read Elliott Eisner's endorsement of my book, "A candid and vivid resource for those wishing to bring about enduring change," I was not only delighted but quite surprised. I had made passing reference to change in *Beginning with Ourselves* (e.g., "The decision to change is up to you," p. 83), but my intent was to emphasize the importance of self-knowledge as a necessary condition for meaningful change, not the change process itself. So I thought that maybe my topic was change. Potential titles occurred to me: "Change from Inside-out," "Facilitating change through beginning with ourselves," and "Images of change."

The first part of this chapter tells the story of how the topic of renewal emerged to replace the original topic of change. In telling my story, I will describe my experience with each of the puzzle pieces and then tell how they fell together with the emergence of an integrating concept.

Images: The Universal Language

My sabbatical began in Finland where I conducted a three-day workshop, with a dozen graduate students in education at the University of Helsinki. I conducted the workshop in English, which was a third or fourth language for most participants, but they used their native language when communicating in pairs and in small groups. For example, I gave English-language instructions for bringing out their own images, they wrote down their thoughts in their native language, shared the experience with a partner in that language, and then shared the experience in the large group in English. Their work in bringing out their learning style and implicit theories was useful, but it was their work with personal images which provided me with the most valuable source of knowledge and energy for my work.

After the students had brought out their images and shared them in small groups, they returned to the large group to focus on a single image. For example, one participant described a flock of migrating geese, and we each became that image, "living in it" for a few moments, entering into it as intensely as possible. One participant expressed concern that she might not be able to lead the flock in the right direction through the long journey south. Another colleague suggested that in her version of the image, the geese alternated in leading the flock so that responsibility was shared. We then returned to become a part of this newly transformed image. (It should be noted that it does not matter whether geese actually alternate in real life. In imagery, anything is possible!)

Another participant's image, a garden, was the focus of our next session. Each of us entered the garden, taking in its beauty, aroma, and texture. Some colleagues became gardeners tending the flowers, while others became the flowers. After we had each immersed ourselves in our own personal gardens, we shared the experience so that our collective garden became transformed into a new richer garden that we could all enter again.

At the following session, when participants applied their images-into-action through creative problem-solving, they could choose from three images: their own initial image, the migrating geese, or the garden. Working in small groups of three or four, participants each evolved an action plan for application in their work (they were all practitioners as well as doctoral students).

At the conclusion of the workshop, I presented each participant with a fresh red rose. We then stood in a circle taking in the beauty and aroma of our own rose and that of the others as we lived together in our shared garden. This was a powerful moment full of high energy for each of us and for the group as a whole.

It was during my reflections on the Helsinki workshop that I was able to work out how the pieces of the puzzle — images, energy, and action — might fit together. I expressed my reflections in three assumptions which one of my student/colleagues later dubbed "Hunt's Hunch":

1. When we identify our personal images, *we connect* with our personal energy.
2. When we share our images, we *release* our energy.
3. When we apply our shared images, we *transform* our energy into action.

These three assumptions form the first major theme described and documented in Chapters Three, Four, and Five of this book. But there are other puzzle pieces to consider first, and these are the subject of the remainder of this chapter.

Seductive Images and Organizational Realities: The Second Time Around

The next piece of the puzzle I considered can be described by Judith Warren Little's (1984) indelible title, "Seductive images and organizational realities," since it highlights the necessity of organizational support for renewal. I had acknowledged the importance of Little's article earlier (Hunt, 1987), but it took on new meaning for me after returning from Finland and conducting a series of workshops primarily with people from the same organization. Briefly I will describe this experience in relation to the emergence of my focus on personal renewal.

Upon returning from Helsinki, I worked with three organizations: a small school board embarking on a board-wide program of active learning, a secondary school initiating a program of integrating handicapped students into all classes, and a newly created career center which had been designed to bring together secondary students' school experience with the world of work. In all three cases, my aims were (1) to demystify the espoused program goals so that participants could connect the project with their past work experience and (2) to evoke personal images (based on their earlier related experiences) which could be shared with colleagues and applied to their present situation.

I began working on the board-wide initiative on active learning by giving a half-day workshop with the principals of the secondary schools, the vice-principals, and department heads. Secondary school staff often consider active learning inappropriate for their students because they erroneously interpret it to mean physical action, requiring that students move around the classroom. Therefore, I began with a short version of the "Identifying your own learning style" exercise in order to encourage participants to bring out the characteristics of a positive learning situation that they had experienced. Next, I proposed a definition of active learning as learning experiences in which students participated actively in their learning through the activity of their minds, feelings, and/or actions. Participants then described characteristics of active learning in their own words. Finally, I asked them to consider the characteristics of their own positive learning experiences and to underline those which fit their definition of active learning. It was an Inside-out introduction to the topic.

The next phase began with participants identifying a positive professional experience in which they had used their own principles of active learning. Participants began to evoke images of active learning through completing sentences such as "Letting my imagination go, this experience reminds me of. . . ." We also used a guided imagery exercise. Next, we shared images and, as in Helsinki, each attempted to enter into a single image. One image of active learning, for example, was a group of writers preparing a script for a TV comedy. To the surprise of many, becoming this image produced additional characteristics of active learning: being non-judgmental, being willing to share and to take risks, and so on. Most participants left with a more accepting, and open, approach to the concept of active learning and its possible practical value.

Two weeks later, I conducted a full-day workshop with 125 secondary school teachers from the same board. I used much the same approach but with far fewer positive results. Although the teachers went through the workshop activities, the energy was lacking. It was not until we began to discuss the next steps for initiating active learning in their classrooms that I discovered that there were in effect no plans for allowing time for teachers to meet together in departmental groups to share and plan their approach. It was expected that they would plan to "implement" the program on their own time through reading the guidelines. There was no organizational support in place for their continuing this activity. Putting myself in their place, I could immediately understand their reluctance to become involved in bringing out their images. Since they had not become actively involved learners themselves, it was very unlikely they would encourage their students to do so. Visions of Judith Warren Little's paper filled my head. No organizational support, no images.

The second example, working with 25 selected secondary teachers in a school initiating a program of integrating disabled students into all classes, provides a similar, though slightly more positive story of working with personal energy in an institutional setting. I began this workshop by inviting participants to focus on their experiences with teaching students of widely varying abilities, specifically inviting them to recall positive experiences in meeting this challenge, and bringing out images from this experience. In the afternoon, when we applied their images to their concerns, I noticed that most of their concerns were not with the students, but about what the new role of the resource teachers would be. I discovered that many of the teachers felt themselves being unfairly burdened with students who had previously been taught by resource teachers. As in the first example, no arrangements had been made for follow-up or for time to share and apply the new initiative. Organizational realities were again at issue. (One year later, I heard informally that this program had gradually been initiated, and that several of the participating teachers felt the workshop had been helpful.)

Finally, I worked with a staff of nine professionals in a newly created career center which had been designed to co-ordinate the resources of the school board with local industry, private foundations, and the federal government in order to bring the school experience in line with the world of work. Since most staff members were new to the project, the half-day workshop was aimed at team building. Their personal images about the project were very rich and valuable. Images such as baking a special cake, giving birth, mountain climbing came quickly, and provided a base for sharing and applying. Because some staff members did not know each other well, the exchange of images provided an especially meaningful, unintrusive way to become aware of one another's deeply held beliefs. Since personal images emanate from our central values and beliefs (Figure 2), I concluded the workshop by suggesting that the value of images is best realized when they are regarded as sources of energy and wisdom to be tapped when difficulties are encountered. The staff response to this initial workshop was very favorable, but, largely due to the enormous demands of launching a new setting, no follow-up occurred to sustain the continuing application of images.

Understanding how organizational support fits into the puzzle turned out to be a challenge — indeed, I still have not fit it in completely, though I have made some progress, described in Chapter Six. My dilemma can be depicted as follows. In negotiating participation in the initiatives described above, I introduced my ideas in the following way:

> As you know, we live in a time when the resources within our organizations are being steadily decreased. We are asked to do more with fewer resources, whether financial, physical, or human. Yet we have an untapped reservoir of resources within. I find that when we respect experienced practitioners and allow them to bring out their inner wisdom, they provide many new ideas, support for one another, creative perspectives, and so on. Yet we rarely take advantage of this resource, relying instead on outside "experts" whose presence may even be stifling.

Inevitably, this statement was greeted with attentive interest on the part of administrators and decision makers who were looking for ways to deal with what Sarason has called "the myth of unlimited resources" (1972). However, when I continued with the next steps in my negotiation, I encountered resistance:

> The inner wisdom and experienced knowledge of experienced staff members are precious human resources which, you have agreed, can become valuable organizational assets. However, it is not enough to bring out these resources; they must be allowed to "flow." It is not sufficient to locate water power; we must establish conditions by which it creates power. In the case of the human resources within organizations, we need to re-arrange priorities, schedules, and timetables so that staff members can meet together on a regular basis to provide resources for one another. Otherwise, their resources will dry up, and identifying them will have no practical value. This means, specifically, that time must be allocated for teachers to meet together to deal with professional concerns by utilizing their shared experienced knowledge.

One administrator informed me that releasing teachers from their regular timetable for such a pursuit was a great idea (implying that it was a great "academic" idea) but that in the real world it was impossible. I was unable to carry my point by indicating that in the real word professional burnout is occurring because of our failure to respect the need for replenishment![2]

I can often plot the development of my ideas through making up new transparencies to be used in my workshops. Here is my most recent overhead.

Practitioners' experienced knowledge: An untapped resource.
Tapping this resource requires:

1. Climate supportive of beginning with ourselves,
2. Time and opportunity to share and apply, and
3. Long term commitment.

---

2. At least I am in good company, for my experience is a clear example of the intractability of the school system which is the key concept in Seymour Sarason's critique, *The Predictable Failure of Educational Reform* (1990a).

Placing these words on a transparency could not, however, sustain my Little Optimist so it was fortunate that at about the same time I received a call from Dr. Helen Hartle, Director of In-Service Training and the Teacher Center Program in New York State, inviting me to present my ideas to their annual conference. I had always felt that teacher centers, as they emerged in the sixties in England, represented ideal organizational support for an Inside-out approach and I referred to them in *Beginning with Ourselves* as "informal, voluntary, grass-roots, practical and fun" (p. 36). So I was delighted to accept Helen's invitation. My half-day plenary workshop with these 400 teacher center colleagues was a peak professional experience for me. Not only were they enthusiastic about the value of personal images, but they also assured me that this important program was indeed providing the necessary organizational support for teacher-centered professional development. As a result, I vowed to make my first post-sabbatical priority raising the awareness of Ontario educators about the value of teacher centers (Hunt, 1989). Although I had not been successful in coping with organizational realities on my own, it was encouraging to discover the potential of teacher centers, which I discuss more fully in Chapter Six.

Change: An Elusive Concept

As my sabbatical approached its half-way point, I felt that the pieces of the puzzle, especially the relationship between internal and external factors, were beginning to fall into place. The internal relationship between personal images and energy remained in the center, and the continuous flow of internal energy required an external factor, organizational support. But I was still uncertain about the place of the concept of change in depicting these relationships.

I struggled with this elusive concept, recalling Lewin's stinger "If you want to understand something, try to change it" and Sarason's book *The Culture of the School and the Problem of Change* (1982), and I was still uneasy. I tried concocting some stingers of my own: "Change begins in here, not out there" and "If you want to facilitate change, you must be willing to change yourself," but I was also haunted by other sayings such as "Change for change's sake" and "The more things change, the more they stay the same." As I tried to deal with these contradictions, I recalled with some amusement that the year before I had received an invitation to participate in a national conference of counselors on the theme, "The more things change, the more they stay the same." This topic was to be the subject of a debate, and the organizers asked which side I wished to defend. I replied that I did not believe that it was a suitable topic for a debate, and we wound up debating a different topic. But the distraction was short-lived. I was stuck on the concept of change. And I was also concerned about how I could make my case for the value of personal images in releasing and transforming energy. I had seen workshop participants become energized and I had recorded their positive reactions, but I had no direct evidence of their experience.

So I hit upon an idea to help me with both problems: I turned to my own "support group," a small group of colleagues who meet informally every two weeks to discuss educational issues. This Educational Development Discussion Group exemplifies continuity since we have been meeting bi-weekly for several years. However, we had ceased meeting this year because of my sabbatical. I proposed to members of the "Thursday Group" that they might benefit from attending some workshops I had been developing, while I would benefit by their agreeing to record their process during the workshops as well as by responding to questions about the concept of change. Their reactions were heartwarming: they were eager to reassemble, had missed our meetings, and were quite happy to help me in whatever way they could.[3]

I had developed a new workshop, "Images of Change," which I hoped would provide me with what I needed to move along on my plans for the book. In preparing the overhead transparencies, I first placed the title "Images of Change" at the top of the page and the *Beginning with Ourselves* logo beneath the title. When it was completed, I realized it looked like a book jacket design, and I thought jokingly to myself: I have the cover for my new book, now if I can get some endorsements to put on the back cover, all I have to do is fill in what goes between. One of the workshop transparencies pinpointed the need for organizational support. Another distinguished between Change from Inside-out and Change from Outside-in:

Change from Outside-in	Change from Inside-out
Implementation models	Practitioner initiated
Mission statements	Local planning
Strategic planning models	Beginning with ourselves

I began the workshop by going through the overheads and discussing the stingers reviewed in Chapter One. We then spent some time on the distinction between Inside-out and Outside-in. Participants were invited to respond to the question, "If you were about to read a book on the topic of change, what would be the major issues/questions you would want the author to address?" I hoped that by addressing their specific questions, I could get back on track in writing about change.

---

3. I appreciate the support of the following colleagues who participated in the workshop: Bill Alexander, Liz Burge, Peter Chisholm, Doreen Cleave-Hogg, Pat Doyle, Patricia Kirby, Solveiga Miezitis, Terry Miosi, the late Michael Orme, Mary Ann Pathey, Ruth Pike, Michael Skolnik, Richard Tiberius, Nancy Watson, and Linda Williams.

The remainder of the first session was devoted to evoking images of change specifically related to an important professional or personal change. (See Appendix 3 for "Images of change.") Next, participants shared their images, first in pairs, then in groups of four, and finally in the total group of sixteen. The process differed from a typical workshop in that participants wrote down their process of bringing out and sharing in detail and made their descriptions available to me. I also tape-recorded some of this process. In the second session, we discussed the initial process and did some application of images into action.

The participants' response to my interest in the topic of change was comprehensive and challenging. I summarize what they conveyed to me as follows:

1. What is the domain of change? Personal, professional, organizational, or educational?
2. Who is the object of change? Self or other? A relationship? An individual or organization?
3. Who initiates change? Is it voluntary or involuntary? Planned or unplanned?
4. How is it characterized or measured and by whom?
   a. As event (outcome) or process?
   b. How is it different from development, adaptation, change in response?
   c. How do we distinguish enduring, meaningful change from trivial?
5. How are internal (personal) and external (organizational) factors facilitated? How do these same factors prevent change from being co-ordinated?
6. Is it possible to change without reference to others or to external circumstances?

These questions were daunting, but even more challenging was the image which the topic of change elicited for one of my "Thursday Group" colleagues, Michael Skolnik:

> A beautiful (and ordinary) rose. A red rose. Authentic. Being what it is. Not trying to be blue because that's trendy or some people like blue. Not trying to conceal or lose its thorns. Not trying to grow a shield from the wind. But standing there, vulnerably being itself. Simple message: be what you are, enjoy being who you are. You don't have to change. You are beautiful as you are.

The Red Rose of Helsinki had re-emerged in the Thursday Group workshop to remind me of the folly of "Change for change's sake," of the need for authenticity, of remaining true to oneself. "Images of Change" was a fine topic for a workshop, but it was not the right topic for my book. I had gone as far as I could alone with my topic, and it was only when I arranged to share my struggle with my Educational Development colleagues that I was able to break through to the discovery of my topic. I have only recently realized that this is an example *par excellence* of the vital role of sharing in the release of energy.

Renewal: The Right Topic

It took me eight months of my Sabbatical to discover what I wanted to write about, and that may seem too long for what seems to be such a simple task. For my part, I felt fortunate that it had not taken much longer because I had found that I could not rush the process. When I try to reconstruct the specific process of switching topics from change to renewal, it is very difficult to know whether I first dropped the idea of change and later discovered renewal, or if renewal came first and replaced change; it probably does not matter. What counts is that I knew it was the right topic. It is tempting to say that the concept of renewal emerged suddenly, allowing all of the pieces of the puzzle to fall into place, but that is not quite true. In coming to the topic, I also came to accept that a part of how it came to me as a topic will always remain beyond analysis and logic.

My initial sense of rightness about the topic came from intuitive feelings. I did not realize, for example, that a logical definition of renewal was implicit in my assumptions about imagery: connecting with our energy, releasing it, and transforming it into action. This definition came much later. Shifting to renewal averted the increasingly complex questions posed by the concept of change, and this was certainly a relief. This was not to say that I would never use the word "change" again, for it is impossible to portray human affairs without it. But I would use it in a more specific sense which would be contrasted with renewal. With my relief there was also a sense of excitement about exploring the territory of renewal. The challenge seemed to bring the possibility of continuous discovery rather than daunting impossibility.

Viewing the Red Rose as an image of renewal rather than of change evoked for me other very affirming images as well. The rose is renewed through the cycle of the seasons, by the soil, water, and sun, by natural rather than prescriptive forces. The renewal of the rose is continuous, ongoing; through renewal, the rose is true to itself.

The closest I can come to putting into words my experience of the rightness of my topic is to emphasize that the idea of renewal provided a rich confirmation of my own experience during my sabbatical year. For example, personal renewal requires organizational support, and in my case I was fortunate in having complete support from OISE to spend my sabbatical in pursuit of self-discovery and the understanding of human affairs. Renewal requires sharing, as I discovered when I became stuck working alone only to be freed through sharing my ideas with my Educational Development colleagues. I had indeed been renewing myself.

Renewal Versus Planned Change

In this section, I emulate Gardner (1982) and Waterman (1987) in attempting to distinguish renewal from change. To do this, I portray renewal as an Inside-out approach, characterized by the "New Three R's" (Hunt, 1987), while I portray planned change as an Outside-in approach (see Table 3). While this contrast may be slightly exaggerated, it provides a framework for discussing differences in greater detail. My critique of planned change might apply equally to the term "reform" (Sarason, 1990a).

Table 3
Renewal Versus Planned Change

Renewal (Inside-out)	Planned change (Outside-in)
1. Begins "in here" (Reflexive)	1. Begins "out there" (Objective)
2. Shared (Reciprocal)	2. Delivered (Unilateral)
3. Ongoing, continuous (Responsive)	3. Put in place (Fixed)

1. Renewal is reflexive; it begins "in here"

The First R, *R*eflexivity, is borrowed from George Kelly's (1955) Reflexivity Principle. It applies to every person and to every situation involving renewal. In professional development, it applies to the facilitator as well as to the participants. I have revised my earlier stinger to reflect my shift in topic from "If you want to facilitate change, you must be willing to change yourself" to "If you wish to facilitate renewal in others, you must begin by renewing yourself." As I proposed in "How to Be Your Own Best Researcher" (Hunt, 1987, pp. 119-121), research-as-renewal begins "in here" with researchers becoming the first participants, experiencing their methods directly before using them to observe others, as elaborated in Chapter Seven. In training-as-renewal, trainers begin by going Inside-out to bring out their own experience in order to evoke their implicit theories and images of training. Before beginning any new experience — a class, a conference, a counseling or consulting session — try to go Inside-out to connect with your own experienced knowledge, especially your images, to guide you in your next professional challenge.

2. Renewal is reciprocal; it needs to be shared

One of the major modifications in my workshops during the past few years has been to increase the opportunity of participants for sharing. In doing so, I try to acknowledge the tension between private reflection and "going public" with a partner by indicating that sharing is optional (Hunt, 1987, p. 82). Nonetheless, my own experience has led me to believe that no one can go it alone. The second R, *R*eciprocality, provides many benefits. In the initial stage of self-discovery, it is reassuring to discover that others experience similar uncertainty as they take up the risk of going Inside-out. At later stages, sharing often amplifies and extends one's experienced knowledge in ways I describe in Chapter Four. As I discovered in my own journey, sharing can help you find your way back when you are lost. Finally, reciprocality is the fundamental basis for the creative problem-solving approach described in Chapter Five.

In teaching, reciprocality consists of working and learning together. In program initiation and training-as-renewal, it involves sharing ideas and developing plans mutually. In research-as-renewal, it involves the researcher and participants joining forces as co-investigators in exploring the terrain together. Such reciprocality is both intellectually supporting and energy enhancing. Sharing is essential in releasing and sustaining the flow of energy, as I will show in portraying cycles of renewal in the final section.

All of this contrasts sharply with the idea of "delivering" services which when you consider its depersonalized implications views the recipient as a helpless pawn.

3. Renewal is responsive; it is ongoing and continuous

The Third R, *R*esponsiveness, reminds us of the quality of "ongoingness" (Van Cauwerberghe, 1988). When the Third R is lost, energy is drained and is not easy to regain. This contrasts sharply with the idea of "putting the program in place." Again, the phrase is extremely revealing when you consider its implications.

If you think of program success as something that is achieved when the program is "in place," then you must ask, What happens next? Will it stay in place by itself? Does it sustain itself? I am not simply engaging in word-play here, but attempting to stimulate thought about the unacknowledged implications of planned change. For example, if you think of programs as being successfully put "in place," then it should not be surprising that once the first program is thought to be "in place," then it will be time to "plug in" another program, and another, and another. Computer programs can be put in place, but not human transactions because energy is required for practitioners to initiate and sustain their responsiveness. I am quite aware of the political appeal of espousing that programs are "in place," even though they may be "non-events," but we should not expect any improvement, or even maintenance, of the quality of practice in education, human services, or health services as long as the role of the practitioner is viewed as putting one program after another "in place." If you are a practitioner, you know all too well the frustration of being required to "implement" a new program before the last one has even been initiated.

This Third R in renewal also reminds us that knowledge is a process, a point with important implications for evaluating and characterizing programs. When evaluators begin to ask, What are the specific arrangements for supporting the continuous evolution and transformation of programs? or, What is being done to sustain and enhance energy? then those planning programs will necessarily make such arrangements rather than giving them lip service.

Ongoingness is of course closely related to sharing and reciprocality. Creating a setting is one thing (Sarason, 1972); sustaining it is another. Sustaining a setting requires specific regularly scheduled arrangements. In such settings with which I am familiar, explicit arrangements are made for weekly meetings in which all staff get together to discuss necessary transformations in their program and model. This was the case in the Community Treatment Project developed by Marguerite Warren (1966) in which treatment workers and researchers met every Friday afternoon to share and discuss their work and modify the treatment model as required. This was also the case with the Psycho-Educational Clinic created by Seymour Sarason at Yale (1966), where all staff assembled on Friday morning to share and discuss their mutual concerns. In both cases, these ongoing, regularly scheduled dialogues provided a continuous source of energy for staff members which enabled them to continue over a long period of time. Perhaps you can add to these examples.

Imagine if a half-day were scheduled every week for teachers to meet, share, and discuss their work and future plans. The time spent in renewal would energize them and improve their time overall in ways I describe in the next section.

That the New Three R's extend the definition of renewal to include the need for organizational support is indicated in Table 4.

Table 4
The New Three R's and Energy Renewal

New Three R's	Process	Energy	Through
1. Reflexive	Begin with yourself	Connect	Self
2. Reciprocal	Share	Release	Self-other
3. Responsive	Sustain	Transformation into action	Organizational support

Cycles of Renewal

Since I began playing variations on the Kolb Cycle (see Abbey, Hunt, & Weiser, 1985), I have discovered a new variation almost every year: as a creative problem-solving model (Chapter Five), as a guide to research (Chapter Seven), as an interview guide (Chapter Seven), and as a means to facilitate communication. I also developed the exercise for demystifying the cycle and developing our own personal versions as described in Chapter One. Now I find that the Kolb Cycle serves as an ideal means for symbolic representation of the process of renewal because the process it represents is ongoing, continuous, and it provides an apt contrast to the linearity of planned change. Yet I was stymied for some time about how to represent the sharing of persons-in-relation by a symbol which was intended only to depict the experiential learning of an individual. I made an earlier attempt (Hunt, 1987, p. 150) to convert the Kolb Cycle to a transactional mode, but it didn't work very well. Before describing how I developed a cycle of renewal which was true to the New Three R's, I will make a few further comments about the Kolb Cycle.

Beginning with Ourselves concluded with a brief section which summarizes a vital, yet often underplayed, feature of the Kolb Cycle: Begin with Concrete Experience (CE). It is Kolb's way of recommending an Inside-out approach. Beginning with my own direct experience (past or present) has proved invaluable in my teaching, thesis supervision, research, interviewing, and workshops; therefore I felt certain that it would also be essential in representing renewal. But how could the Kolb Cycle be transformed to accommodate sharing, which is central to renewal? The solution came when I juxtaposed the four points on the Kolb Cycle to the four steps involved in bringing out and applying experienced knowledge. (See Table 5.)

Table 5
Kolb Cycle and Experienced Knowledge

Phase in Cycle	Steps in Experienced Knowledge
1. Concrete Experience (CE)	Recall positive experience
2. Reflective Observation (RO)	Bring out knowledge
3. Abstract Conceptualization (AC)	Share knowledge
4. Active Experimentation (AE)	Apply knowledge

If we conceptualize the four steps as a continuous cycle of recalling and applying experienced knowledge, it seems quite natural to use the Kolb framework. Careful readers may say, "Wait a minute — sharing is not a form of Abstract Conceptualization," and they will be technically correct. However, point-to-point equivalence is unnecessary in playing a renewal variation on the Kolb theme. What is necessary is that we extend it to include another person or persons. I achieved the representation of a two-person transaction by depicting the second person in a mirror image, so that the symbol becomes a figure 8, as shown in Figure 3.

Figure 3
Renewal as Persons-in-Relation

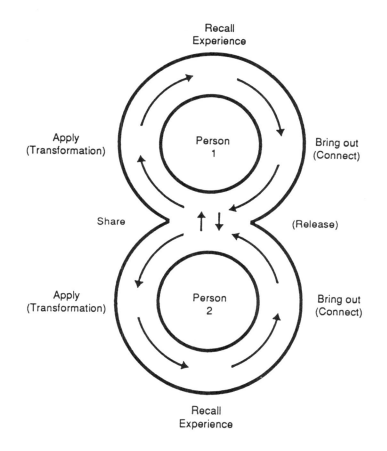

Recall
Experience

Apply
(Transformation)

Person
1

Bring out
(Connect)

Share

(Release)

Apply
(Transformation)

Person
2

Bring out
(Connect)

Recall
Experience

Playing variations on the Kolb Cycle can be contagious. After showing the figure-8 version at a workshop, my host, John Baldry, constructed another variation (Figure 4) to depict renewal as synergy where synergy is defined as the whole (total energy) being greater than the sum of its (energy) parts. Extending Figure 3 to Figure 4 is an excellent example of transformation through sharing.

Perhaps the most striking implication of these two figures is the essential role of sharing in maintaining the flow of energy resources. Let's try to involve you in some more active participation to convey this vital point. Look at Figure 3 and place your finger over the intersection of the two circles to symbolize that sharing has been omitted. What will happen? The energy will cease to flow. It has been identified through bringing out, but it cannot be transformed into action unless it has been *released through sharing.* One might go through the procedure of applying one's knowledge directly (omitting the sharing phase), but such application would be devoid of energy. It is also true that when energy is cut off through omitting the sharing, it cannot be easily switched on again.

All this brings us back to the essential role of organizational support in maintaining and extending the flow of energy resources. Specifically, these cycles of renewal emphasize that support for renewal *must* involve time and opportunity for sharing on a regularly scheduled, long-term basis. The benefits are many, as I will discuss; failure to provide support for renewal can only lead to increasing burn-out. As these "flow charts" show, the synergy of sharing requires openness on the part of individuals and organizations, a point elaborated in Chapter Six which presents the Spirit of Renewal framework. Before developing this framework, I turn in the next three chapters to the relationship between images and energy.

Figure 4
Renewal-As-Synergy

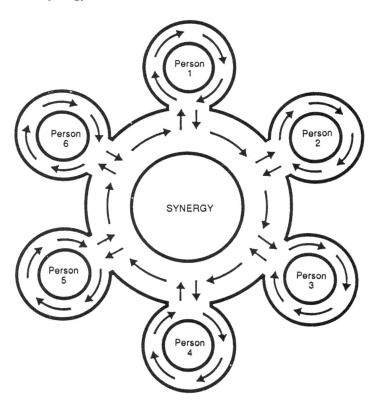

CHAPTER THREE

Personal Images: Connecting with Energy

"Images are the missing link between the mind and the body."
Ken Wilber

The theme of this and the following two chapters is the role of personal images in energy renewal — how they connect us with our energy, release our energy, and transform it into action. This chapter is specifically concerned with identifying our images as this process *connects* us with our energy. I will also describe the characteristics of personal images and distinguish them from similar concepts such as metaphors and symbols. But reading about personal images, "out there," is not enough to appreciate their value for energy renewal; you need to experience them, "in here," within yourself.

Personal images are our inner representations of our experience through our imagination. Some people may feel, "My imagination is very limited, I'm not the artistic type." It is certainly true that imagery is vital to artists, but it is equally true that each of us has an imagination to call on, even though it may be a bit rusty from disuse. You may experience your imagination through memories, hopes, and daydreams, and these offer gateways to your personal images. So I invoke your patience as I invite you to explore your personal images, because I realize that you may not appreciate them until you have completed the chapter. You have nothing to lose by trying out what it is like to trust your imagination. Hundreds of the experienced practitioners with whom I have worked have done so and discovered a new-found resource. I do not promise a source of perpetual renewal and eternal youth, but you may discover something new about yourself and you may even have fun.

I use the term, "personal image," because the experience is "in here," not "out there." An image may be depicted on a printed page, as in the rushing stream described in Chapter One; however, it does not become a personal image until you have made it a part of your inner life, until you have become a part of the image yourself, entering into it with your senses and your imagination.

I begin with a simple exercise for bringing out your own personal image(s), and I hope you are willing to try it. Those of you who need a logical basis before trying something new may want to read ahead to the sections on the characteristics of personal images and on how they differ from symbols and metaphors as well from "outside" images. Those who prefer to learn by reading examples may wish to go to Appendix 4, especially to the images of Kit. If you choose to jump ahead to the rationale or to the example, I hope you will return to the exercise to develop your own experiential foundation for understanding the meaning of personal images.

Identifying Your Personal Images

I invite you to spend a few moments evoking your own personal image(s) so that you will have a first-hand basis for following the discussion. Your first reaction may be that you don't think in images. If so, let me encourage you to consider your daydreaming, your mental activity before and after you do something, and, of course, your dreams. Each of us has our own world of imagery; we simply need to connect with it. For those of you who see no point in actively engaging the topic under consideration, let me ask: Are you interested in finding a new approach to renewing your own personal energy? If you are, why not try the exercise below?

*   *   *

First, identify a positive experience, perhaps the one you used in Chapter One; it can be either a positive professional experience or a positive personal experience. Select an experience which stands out clearly as one in which you felt good about yourself. Don't write it down — just recall it in your memory. When you have selected this specific positive experience, spend a few moments recalling it in more detail. When did it happen? Where did it happen? Make sure that you are in the experience, not just observing it. Allow the experience to fill your senses. What did it look like? What were the sounds, smells, touches? What were your feelings in that moment?

Using these questions as guides, take a few moments to relive the experience as intensely as possible. If you find yourself becoming distracted, focus on your feelings.

*   *   *

Now, come back from re-experiencing the situation. If you have a paper and pen at hand, draw a large circle and then jot down the main features of what you remembered about the experience: qualities, feelings, ideas, what was said; feel free to draw symbols or pictures. If you don't have any paper, or you don't wish to write, go through this process in your mind.

*   *   *

Next, using your associations as a spring-board, complete the following four sentences. Allow yourself to relax and to write down whatever comes to mind in this free association.

1. This experience reminds me of . . .
2. Letting my imagination go, this experience seems like . . .
3. Describing this experience as being like something else, I would say . . .
4. I think of myself as . . .

From your responses, select the one personal image that you prefer and refer to it as we go through the chapter.

At this point, your reaction is probably one of the following:

1. You evoked an image and you are looking forward to exploring it further.
2. You evoked an image, perhaps briefly, but feel uneasy about it either because you are uncertain of its value or its rightness for you.
3. You were unable to evoke an image, and perhaps you feel a bit inadequate.
4. You simply read through the instructions without becoming personally involved in evoking an image.
5. You became aggravated with the request, stopped reading and closed the book. (If you are reading this, welcome back!)

For those of you in the second and third categories, I will describe how others overcame their initial uneasiness. For those of you in the fourth and fifth categories, I will try once more. At least select an image from those we have discussed earlier: a rushing stream, a red rose, a balloon, or perhaps one from Appendix 4.

Thanks for your indulgence. Keep your own image at the ready, as I will refer to it throughout the chapter. I hope that the process of evoking your image not only helps you understand personal images, but also is a first step in your own renewal.

Characteristics of Personal Images

The essence of personal images is their inner meaning to each of us. Therefore, as you read the following characteristics, consider each one as it applies to your own personal image. These characteristics are based partly on the characteristics of experienced knowledge described in Chapter One and partly on comments made by participants as they brought out their personal images.[4]

1. Personal images are unique

Every person's images are like *no* other person's images, to paraphrase Kluckhohn and Murray (1948). Consider the personal image you evoked in the preceding exercise: it may be a familiar one such as a rose, a stream, or a garden. That is, your personal image is in some ways like all other personal images (as I discuss in the next section). Yet your image of a garden, say, is unique because it is your garden and has qualities like no other garden, and it is these distinct qualities that need to be emphasized to bring out the energy potential of the image.

2. Personal images are often unexpressed

Partly because we live primarily in a world which values cognition, logic, and rationality more than imagination, and partly because many of us have become disconnected from our imagination, we rarely bring out and connect with our personal images. Consider your own image and ask yourself, "Have I ever brought out an image like this before?" As one student/colleague put it:

> Focusing on images provides a way to make conscious and deliberate what is often intuitive in our dealings with students and colleagues.

3. Personal images offer new perspectives

When you enter into your image and become a part of it, say living in your garden, this provides a fresh viewpoint. If you enter into your image, do you notice a different world view? A new perspective? A fresh horizon? These images are like new theories in that they direct our attention to relationships we may have overlooked as well as spotlight new relationships:

---

4. All of the images discussed in this chapter as well as the image you identified are *positive* personal images. There are, of course, negative images, e.g. prisoner, but in my experience they have no energy potential. I do not deny the negative, but prefer to use the resources of positive image to address our negative concerns as described in Chapter Five.

Imagery provides an opportunity to unclutter the mind and focus on an image of oneself that reality often obstructs.

4. Personal images may be experienced in all our senses

The dictionary definition of "image" is "a mental representation of anything not actually present to *our senses*" (my italics). Some people equate all images with "visions" and refer to the exercises for bringing out images as exercises in "visualization." Yet personal images are best experienced through all of our senses, and occasionally experienced with no visual quality whatsoever. They are also much more than simply verbal, and may be difficult to render into words. Consider your own image and attempt to extend your experience of it to other modalities: hearing, smelling, tasting, touching, and feeling. The following comments illustrate the multi-sensory quality of personal images:

> The image [that of an invitation to dance] presented itself kinesthetically, visually, and affectively in such a powerful way that there was no doubt of its rightness for me.

> The physical environment [image of a fair] was not very clear but I could hear the screams of delight, feel the crowd pushing all around me, smell the aroma of various foods mingling in the air, and sense the excitement of curious spectators.

> The overriding sense that I experienced was kinesthetic, making contact with the soft cloud, gentle breeze in space, touching others. This was certainly a novel additional element to the teaching experience. The image of a cloud was instrumental in allowing this sensory modality to develop.

Sometimes they may be primarily kinesthetic:

> Waves constantly in motion with ups and downs. Potential for storm: power.

5. Experiencing personal images requires a temporary suspension of critical judgment

Entering the world of imagery requires sending your Critic away temporarily. Put positively, you are invited to become a child again, to connect with your spontaneous, whimsical part and to allow it to come on stage. Each of us must make our own arrangements for leaving our Critic behind, and, for most, it takes a lot of initial patience and practice. Think back to your own experience in bringing out your personal image: Were you aware of the difficulty in becoming non-judgmental? What were you afraid might happen? Did you realize that the suspension of your

Critic is *temporary*, that you can retrieve it whenever you wish (see Hunt, 1990, for a more detailed discussion)? And on a more positive note, did setting your Critic aside lead to experiences which were enjoyable and perhaps surprising? As one colleague put it:

> I need to learn to suspend my critical thinking, and let some of my underlying feelings and creativity into the process.

6. In imagery, anything is possible

Closely related to the last characteristic, we find that personal images do not operate according to the rules of reality. If you do not like an image which comes to you, you can simply tell it to go away. If a personal image seems somehow incomplete, you can ask the image what it needs and transform it. For example, if your image is a garden, you may wish to enhance it by moving it into the sky, or by allowing the plants to communicate with one another. In response to my suggestion that in imagery anything was possible, a student/colleague commented:

> With this new permission, I found myself focusing on my image of a sun ray. Rays began to zoom ahead of me into a lush green forest. The rays brought internal knowledge and life to the growing world.

7. Each of us has a wide repertory of personal images

As you were identifying your own personal image, chances are that you considered more than one. Personal images vary in many ways: their aptness for a particular situation, their closeness to our core beliefs, and our feeling of their "rightness." Consider two or three images which you might have selected in terms of how they feel: Does one seem more appropriate for a work situation than another? Does one feel more personally relevant? Like most questions I am raising here, these will require more time than you wish to devote at the moment, and I will raise them again. Here are some examples of the variety of personal images:

> Later I would find other personal images which would also be useful. I'm at the center of a bubbling spring which also invigorates those around me. The flame I possess — a light which can shine through me; the calm glow in my center that warms and stills me also warms others. Then I can call down a blanket of calm over a situation, a calm which is protective of all. My images are many and useful.

> My images seem to fall into two categories, the first related to my work as a community resource person and the second related to my teaching in a community college.

Group 1	Group 2
Truth seeker	Entertainer
Paulo Friere	Juggler
Jesus's biblical learning	Teapot
	Water sprinkler

8. Each of us can sense the "rightness" of our personal images

Given the variety of the images that we might bring out, how can we decide which one(s) to choose and pursue? As with experienced knowledge, each of us must make the choice; it cannot be made by another. Those of you who are especially self-critical will be thinking that this process requires a return of your Critic. Not so. Pursuing the sense of aptness or relevance of an image is an intuitive process whereby we search for the image(s) most central to our core beliefs. And the closer the personal image to our central beliefs, the stronger the connection to our personal energy. Following is an example:

> My search for an image of my work was an arduous one; initial attempts to develop an image seemed frustrating and fruitless. However, my subconscious must have taken hold of the task, for three images emerged in rough form during one contemplative session out in the summer sun.
> In one image, I see my students as indoor plants — all different shapes, sizes, colors, and needs. I see myself as the indoor gardener, nurturing the plants, watering, feeding, and providing enough light for growth. If I care for them properly, they will flourish.
> The second image to emerge was that of a hot air balloon. In this image, the balloon is the source of learning. My students and I take a journey in the balloon which soars upward as we learn more and more. At times, I am the guide and my students are the travelers, and at other times in the journey we switch roles. It is a continuous journey, punctuated by brief rests as the balloon touches down for refuelling and for new travelers.
> The third image, the strongest one, is that of a campfire. In this image, I am the campfire builder, organizing the fuel and providing the spark for the flames. My classroom is the fire and my students, the flames. As I nurture the fire, it flickers, dances, and grows warmer. The flames grow together to create a powerful whole. I observe it carefully, tending it so that it neither dies out nor burns out of control. I, in turn, enjoy watching the fire develop and I appreciate the beauty of the whole.
> It is the third image that I felt most comfortable with and excited about. As I continued to think about it, I was able to form the image in a more detailed way and it became an aid to developing a greater understanding of my teaching and learning styles.

These characteristics typify personal images which are most likely to connect with our personal energy, a topic discussed in detail at the end of this chapter. Also, I will add to these eight characteristics in the next chapter when I discuss how the shared aspects of personal images contribute to the release of personal energy.[5]

Distinguishing Personal Images from Symbols and Metaphors

Since each person's inner experience is unique, it is not easy to describe it in words. In this section, I discuss why I prefer "personal images" to similar descriptive terms such as "metaphors" and "symbols." In discussing this preference, I do not intend to dictate what language you should use to describe your own inner experience. You may find that your experience is accurately described by the term "symbol" or some other term such as "representational system" (Bandler & Grinder, 1979). But first, I'll take a turn.

My preference for personal images is recent, since I used metaphors earlier (Hunt, 1987). Like the word "image," "metaphor" has been extremely popular in the past few years, spawning many books and even a journal by that title. Most of us first encounter the word "metaphor" in an English course, perhaps learning to distinguish a literary metaphor from a simile, activities requiring our critical faculties. Later, we may have been taught to consider literary metaphors in terms of their evocativeness or richness, again applying critical judgment. Yet the personal value of our images cannot be judged by applying the criteria of literary criticism. For example, consider your own image as it might be viewed for its literary richness, and you will see how applying criteria of literary criticism is inappropriate and unproductive.

This is especially true for frequently occurring personal images such as a rose, a stream, or a garden, which by standards of literary criticism are considered trite. Yet such judgment is premature and cuts off consideration of the potential personal value which can only be determined by experiencing your image and exploring its personal meaning. Your rose is like no other person's rose.

Like "metaphor," the word "symbol" triggers our Critic, but in a somewhat different arena. When we think of a symbol, we may think of its psychoanalytical, or sexual, significance, as indicated by the theory of unconscious dynamics. Many of us have encountered the term "symbol" in Freudian psychoanalysis which, for example, might view a rose as a vaginal symbol. The assumption of sexual symbolic

---

5. See Yabroff (1990) for a similar list of characteristics of "Inner image."

meaning may have value in psychoanalytic treatment, but when entering our own world of imagination, sexual symbols are as inappropriate as literary metaphors. Both "metaphor" and "symbol" rely on Outside-in judgments.

Perhaps the extreme of such preoccupation with the symbolic significance of images is to be found when one uses a Jungian dictionary of the archetypal meaning of symbols. Leaving aside the validity of such "translations" (they certainly reveal a lot about our Outside-in search for meaning), they are completely counter to the spirit of evoking personal images from Inside-out. As noted earlier, it is true that in some ways our personal images are like all other personal images, and this similarity is captured by the collective unconscious and the archetypal significance of symbols. However, to interpret the image of a rushing stream as equivalent to "life force" is not initially helpful. After one has worked with a personal image, shared it, and applied it, there is the possibility that it might be enriched by considering its archetypal significance (an example of reinstating our critical judgment after its temporary suspension), but such consideration of symbolic significance should come much later in the process.

A final reason for preferring personal image as a term is the implication of its arising from our imagination rather than from our unconscious. My invitation to connect with and explore your imagination is intended to demystify the process, to offer a resource which is under your control. By contrast, to connect with your unconscious probably requires the guidance of an expert, if not a psychoanalyst. Personal images come from our imagination, from our fantasies, from our daydreams. Bringing out and experiencing them is possible for everyone. Yet demystifying the process does not imply a lessened respect for their power. Working with our own images or helping others to work with theirs should be done in a spirit of respect for this potency. Images are a powerful source of energy and wisdom. We also need gentleness, and, to some extent, caution so that if we don't like what is happening or do not wish to work with an image, we can simply tell the image to go away.

In summary, leave the metaphors to the literary critics and the symbols to the psychoanalysts. We claim our personal images for ourselves.

Personal Images and Outside Images

Another benefit of bringing out our personal images is that the awareness we gain helps us to see through externally imposed images and to avoid being manipulated by them. Our personal images are such powerful forces in determining our actions that it should be no surprise that image manipulation is a central activity in selling and advertising and in political campaigns. Corporate advertisers and political media "handlers" create images "out there" with the hope that these images will penetrate to the consumer's or voter's inner values and beliefs, and thus influence the decision to buy their product or candidate. Associating a product — or a politician — with a positive image, such as a beautiful beach or a fireside, is intended to evoke your own positive personal images, without your awareness, so that you become more favorable to the product or the politician.

The best way to deal with the constant bombardment of external images is to become aware of your own personal images. This awareness serves as a foundation for counteracting attempts at manipulation. Dealing with image manipulation calls for the return of your Critic. Then, when you watch a TV commercial which features a beautiful beach, you can enjoy it from the inside while dissociating it from the product. Awareness of our own personal images therefore not only boosts our confidence and provides us with an internal anchor, but it is also a base for freeing us from external manipulation (more about this in Chapter Eight).

External images are not always used for manipulation, and may be turned to our advantage as long as we consider them in relation to our own personal images, or use them in a way that is Inside-out rather than Outside-in. For example, it may be useful to consider the Outside-in categories of images which Fox puts forward in "Personal Theories of Teachers" (1983) or which Morgan develops in *Images of Organization* (1986). In both cases, the authors provide a variety of categories of images which may enhance your own personal images and raise your awareness of others.

Fox (1983) suggests four categories of teachers' theories/images: (1) shaping theories in which the teacher molds the student, (2) transfer theories in which the teacher relays information directly to the student, (3) traveling theories in which teacher and student are both on a journey, and (4) growth theories in which the teacher facilitates the development of the student. Fox describes each of these categories in detail (see Hunt, 1987, p.81), including the verbs associated with each category.

In *Images of Organization* (1986), Gareth Morgan describes a variety of images from an Outside-in perspective. Organizations are depicted as (1) machines, (2) organisms, (3) brains, (4) cultures, (5) political systems, (6) psychic prisons, and (7) places for transformation. These categories permit (1) a comparison of the similarities between your personal image and the image of your organization, and (2) an orientation to your organization in terms of potential support for renewal (see Chapter Six).

Just as there are many varieties and sources of images, so there are many purposes of imagery. Evoking and experiencing personal images as discussed here is only one of the many uses of imagery and imagination. Applications of imagery have increased enormously during recent years in a variety of areas and purposes: reducing phobias, sports psychology, overcoming anxieties, coping with life-threatening illness, and acquiring interpersonal skills. My use of imagery is, specifically, to evoke images which can later be applied to professional and personal concerns. You may find other uses of imagery valuable as well, but here we focus on evoking your personal images.

Creating the Climate for Evoking Personal Images

In responding to instructions, many people find it difficult to relinquish temporarily their "mind focus" or to suspend their critical judgment. Taking on a non-judgmental attitude of openness is not so easy as it sounds and is often considered risky. Therefore, in my workshops, I try to create an environmental tone which will encourage this shift: I play soft, relaxing music and I often leave a summary of suggestions for going Inside-out on each participant's chair. The suggestions include the following:

1. Send your Critic away.
2. Don't worry about going public — write for yourself.
3. Try to bring out what is, not what should be.
4. Remember, self-knowledge is the first step toward change.
5. But also remember that the choice is up to you.

(Hunt, 1987, pp. 82-83)

Because connecting with our imagination requires an inner climate of patience, gentleness, and openness, I often compare beginning to experience our imagination with beginning a regime of physical fitness. Most of you have probably embarked on a routine of physical exercise at some time, and chances are you initially found your body a little rusty from disuse. Easing into a regime of physical exercise calls for gentleness to your body, patience in not expecting immediate results, and openness to the possibilities of communicating with your body. If you were committed to respecting your body while maintaining your patience, gentleness, and openness, then you probably found that gradually you became aware of your body, your heart rate, and your breathing rate. It is likely, too, that through this regime, you came to experience your body as an integral part of your whole self, not a mechanism removed from your mind and feelings. The same is true for your imagination. To give personal images a chance, you need to adopt the same orientation — gentleness, patience, and openness, and spend time connecting with this important part of yourself.

Patience is especially important for persons who are just re-connecting with their imagination after many years of disuse. So don't expect dramatic images to present themselves immediately. Like anything worthwhile in life, it will take time and commitment. The qualities of gentleness, patience, and openness gradually evolve into the most central quality: self-trust.

Approaches for Bringing Out Personal Images

Free association

The exercise at the beginning of the chapter is an example of using free association to evoke personal images. It involves identifying a specific event, recalling it for a few moments, jotting down your associations to the event (including non-verbal associations), and then responding to incomplete sentences which are intended to stimulate your imagination.

I often use free association to introduce a workshop or even a conference. Free association is relatively non-threatening and provides a first step into the world of imagination. It may evoke images which come from your Critic, that is, what you think you should imagine, rather than from your imagination, but this is still a first step, and your Critic may be gradually suspended. For those who are so disconnected from their imagination that they cannot evoke an image through free association, I suggest that they simply "borrow" one from a list (Appendix 4).

From our language

We may reveal our personal images through our choice of words (Bandler & Grinder, 1979; Fox, 1983; Mumby, 1985). Even though we are unaware of this influence, we may speak of *"moving along," "getting stuck,"* and being *"almost there"* without realizing we are using the language of an inner journey. Each of the personal theories and organizational images of Fox and Gardner in the last section have associated language which reveals the underlying image. Identifying our personal images from our language requires tape-recording our speech or writing a journal so that we can reflect on the language of our innermost thoughts and feelings.

Guided imagery

Guided imagery is the method *par excellence* for evoking personal images. Appendix 1 includes a verbatim transcript of a guided imagery exercise. In introducing guided imagery, I try to demystify the concept by indicating that its meaning, as implied by its name, involves guiding people to connect with their imagination. I compare guided imagery with physical fitness, as described above, and emphasize that what occurs is completely under the individual's control so that if something occurs which he or she doesn't like, it can simply be dismissed. In imagery, anything is possible. It may often require two or three imagery sessions for participants to trust the process, but eventually images present themselves. Although guided imagery need not be mystical, it is a powerful method and needs to be respected as such. It is similar to hypnosis in that it invites relaxation and provides guidance as one tries to connect with non-conscious levels of the self; however, as I use guided imagery, participants are made aware in advance of what I will say and told they are in control if they want to send an image away.

The rest of this chapter largely consists of reflective comments from student/ colleagues in my Learning Styles class. Their experiences typify issues and concerns that arise as we experiment with ways to bring out our personal images. The first comments from a student/colleague address the difference in image evoked by free association and by guided imagery:

> We developed two images, one by free association and one by guided imagery. The image I developed through free association was of an experienced guide leading the students on an exploration, providing the kind of help they needed to complete the trip. The destination was set and my role was to help them select the right maps, learn to read them, use equipment appropriately, and so on. They were the ones who *took* the trip but I also learned from them.
>   The image from the guided imagery exercise was of my students and myself at a race track, cheering on our winning horse. The atmosphere was electric, full of good feelings and excitement. We were comrades pulling together for the same goal.
>   Perhaps it was the nature of the two exercises that created the focus on different aspects of my teaching experience. An image which would be most useful in grounding my practice would include both components, and reflect their integration.

The following comments illustrate how two participants in the exercises moved away from their initial uneasiness in the process to a sense of trust, movement made possible by their "letting go":

> Bringing out my personal images was relatively new to me. But the preparation of breathing, relaxing, clearing, and centering was very helpful. We were then invited to sense the sights, sounds, and tactile stimuli. Soon I found that an image of a radiant silver moon presented itself. From that moment on, I felt relaxed about guided imagery — realizing that an image would emerge if I relaxed and let it happen.

*   *   *

> Not having participated in imagery exercises previously, I felt uneasy. I did not

know if I was on the right track or if my image was meaningful. I wasn't sure *what* to imagine. But then I quickly realized that imagery has no language of its own — one must experience it. A part of me remained detached at first. Once I let go, I really got into it.

Following are four more extended comments from student/colleagues about their process of searching for their images:

This was the most difficult task for me. I really didn't receive a clear image during guided imagery. Then I saw a light shining into a globe-shaped crystal. I also saw that the crystal was the head of the boy I was teaching in my positive teaching experience. From this image I have since developed my image of teaching. I like my image. The dancing spectrums produced by crystals create both beauty and movement.

I had been very anxious to develop a suitable image. A year ago, a teacher retired from our school after having spent most of her adult life teaching, and finished the last few years of her career as our school's guidance counsellor. I think I'll hear her voice forever exhorting all teachers to make their classrooms a "safe harbor" for students. Her message put into words what I already realized — that for an increasing number of students school may be the only safe place from emotional, racial, or even physical attack. I tried to develop a "harbor master" image from the emotional commitment her words had given me.

I know I'll use my harbor master image whenever I feel hollow or impatient, but I like my "crystals" image better. I believe that I am a lifelong student, exposing different aspects of myself to new learning experiences. I hope that I can instill in my students a joy for learning so it becomes a lifetime avocation for them as well.

*   *   *

My first image of a positive professional experience, that of a hostess at a garden party, arose when I was reflecting on a positive experience as an HRD [Human Resource Development] practitioner. At first, it did not seem to fit my matching style with my students. But today, reflecting on what I have written so far, I feel that the hostess image fits my matching with my students. For example, if a guest cannot eat certain foods, a thoughtful hostess will make sure alternatives are provided which are just as nutritious and as beautifully presented. As a teacher, I try to offer my students choices or alternatives to suit them. A hostess is also very careful to foster harmony and understanding among all her guests, just as I attempt to do among the students in my class. A hostess also wants to provide her guests with opportunities to exchange views and ideas. Again, I see myself doing this in my classroom.

*   *   *

The image of a very large, beautiful beech tree was the next image to emerge, and became very compelling for me. The tree stands beside a pond with a waterfall; there is grass all around, flowers, and a clump of smaller beech trees. The branches are filled with birds of every color and type. They are singing, eating, feeding younger birds, learning to fly — all are making a busy, noisy sound. The birds create great energy, and there is a lot of wind and energy swirling through my branches. Sometimes the tree wishes for winter so the birds will fly away for a while and the tree can rest for a time. I am the beech tree. I am nurturing and protective. If my roots were not so strong and deep, at times I might fear being blown over. . . . The birds are my students. They get what they want from me and from each other. Some get different things. The smaller trees are the new teachers whom I bend over to help.

This image was very powerful and liberating for me. I had never attempted guided imagery before, and I had to experience and then discard two other images before accepting the beech tree image. Exploring it with a partner was a very rewarding experience. I am not used to revealing much about myself, but I felt very safe in this situation.

*   *   *

Initially, I found it difficult to let any kind of image emerge; I seemed to be restless and unable to relax. (I know I was stressed out because of a very busy day at school.) Perhaps my aching back prevented me from finding a comfortable posture. Eventually I put my head down on the table, and tried to doze — not a real sleep, but just relaxing in that "twilight" zone. Then the images started to flow. The one that stayed was that of collecting shells. The image was a powerful one for me — I found it to be refreshing and energizing.

*   *   *

With the introduction of the guided imagery session, I began to feel some anxiety as I had previously tried out such an exercise and found it frustrating and uneventful. I found as I was trying to relax and clear my mind all sorts of interference from my previously "cooked" images came rushing to the forefront. At the same time, I felt of this sort of activity was "hokey."

The instructions to envision the place and the feelings associated with a positive learning experience helped me to become refocused. I found myself mentally walking through the building and then walking outside of the perimeter. A coiled garden hose flashed in my mind and began to uncoil as if it were a living being and to wrap itself around and through the windows of the three-story building that I had envisioned in my mind. My initial reaction to this incident was one of dismissal as I tried to erase the bizarre vision from my mind. Within seconds I began to realize that a garden hose had never been at the place I was revisiting in my mind and I decided to call the strange image back again. The hose seemed to represent reality and adaptability to warm sunshine, to harsh cold, etc.

*   *   *

Sometimes, the image presents itself when we least expect it:

I spent considerable time in thinking about an image that would sit well with me. I thought through two or three that I could have used, but each did not leave me feeling satisfied. As I was continuing to think through this on my back porch, my eyes settled on several cocoons on the overhang of the roof.

Immediately my image began to present itself, slowly at first, and then faster and faster, as my mind started racing with words and pictures like an exploding kaleidoscope.

Becoming and Living Your Image

Evoking your personal image is not sufficient to connect you with your personal energy; you need to experience it. Participants give different descriptions of this process: becoming your image, living in your image, entering into it, exploring your image, and so on. Whatever words you use, the process is essential to connecting with your energy. Becoming and entering into your image may not come easily at first. It requires practice, trust, and patience.

Let's try a brief exercise. Recall the image you evoked earlier, then allow yourself to enter into it, to become a central part of it. If for any reason you find it difficult to become part of your image, remember that in imagery anything is possible and make arrangements so that you can live in your image for a time. Make certain that you are *in* the image, a part of it, not observing the image from outside. As you enter into it, pay attention to your feelings, senses, and perceptions. How does it feel? Allowing your feelings expression is vital to becoming the image. How does the world seem from that perspective? What do you see? Hear? Smell? Here are a few other questions to consider.

1. Where are you in the image?
2. How do you feel?
3. What makes the image go?
4. What does it need?
5. Where are the others in the image?
6. How are you related to the others?

It is not easy to explore your image on your own, and in the next chapter I describe how this exploration is facilitated by working with a partner.

Following are excerpts from a student/colleague's experience:

At first I was conducting the first movement of Beethoven's Sixth Symphony. I saw the instruments and heard them play. I really wanted this image but it quickly gave way to a field of flowers with the music playing in the background. Gradually, the image focused on a cluster of flowers and there was a bee going from flower to flower, pollinating each one.

I asked the bee, "Who could you be?" [dialoguing in the image]

The bee said, "I am you. I pollinate the flowers, your clients, with warmth, love, and intimacy."

Then I asked, "What do I need?" and the reply was the same, "Warmth, love and closeness."

Then he presented a gift — a jar of honey and the sun. As I became the bee, I collected pollen from some of the flowers and returned it to others in the form of empowerment. I am related to the others since I need the pollen for food (development and growth). The image needs the flowers and the pollen to keep growing. It also needs the ebb and flow of the wind and the music.

Does Becoming Your Image Connect You With Your Energy?

Since developing this idea I have tried to collect information on its validity by inviting student/colleagues in my Learning Styles class to respond to the following question: "As you brought out and became your image, were you aware of connecting with your energy? If so, describe it as specifically as possible. If not, what was your experience?"

First, I include responses from those whose examples have been used earlier:

The stream:

> I definitely connected both with the image and the feelings/energy it generated. In becoming the stream, I was able to feel the bubbling effervescence of the water, the eagerness to forge on ahead. I was also very aware of the fulfilling feeling in joining with other streams — and of a sense of loss as they once again went on their way. My final visualization was almost of a torrent — rushing and swelling. I experienced a heady sense of power, of newness, a feeling I could go anywhere, do anything. This gave me a sense of affirmation, of strength. I also felt a need to control my journey, despite its speed. The presence of water — of myself as water — was soothing and refreshing. All those blues and greens.

The bubble:

> I relate to the image of a bubble because it is full of energy and ideas. It explodes into many other bubbles, and they have energy; they also have the desire to share their energy and ideas. The bubble is the source of energy. It gives off energy. The image is alive. I feel that my image reflects me because I tend to be a very energetic person. I like to feel positive and enthusiastic in most things that I do.

The sun ray:

> As I became my image my energy seemed to be released. I felt a freeing up of myself. My rays took on a more flexible form. I felt freedom from my restrictions — and the rays travelled into the forest encircling the trees, plants

and animals. I have not put myself into the complete feeling of the speed that I see because I fear speed. Though I'm very much a "here and now" "concrete experience" person, I tend to avoid sensations that I fear. But I do *see* my rays zigzagging and thrusting. I do feel the warmth, and the light that I bring. The feeling of speed — the energy, the exhilaration needs to be explored.

The bee:

I was aware of connecting with my energy when I brought out and became my image. I felt a jolt of energy, just like electricity, which started at my feet and moved through my body and made me jump from my chair. I felt somewhat excited as I went to explore my image.

Here are some others:

In my image [the canoe/wilderness trip], I felt that I definitely connected with my energy. Energy *is* the essence of my image. Energy is abundant, everything consists of energy: the water, grass, soil, rocks, rotting logs. The wind/air as it surrounds us is energy — energy that we absorb into our being. Energy that allows us to go on and on. It felt so good, so warm and powerful, so life-giving. Nothing prickly about this energy — no pain, no jolts, no off-color flashes. Go ahead, try it! Put your hand in the water and absorb the energy. Feel the warmth and goodness of the flow. Feel the color. Feel the power. Feel the beauty, how pure and dynamic. Feel yourself becoming energized.

*   *   *

As I became my image [a bird], I was aware of the tremendous energy required to lift off the ground to become airborne. Once in flight my energy was restored as I soared effortlessly, buoyed by the power of the wind. I felt warmth and lightness and these seemed to restore my energy as did the peacefulness and freedom of flight.

*   *   *

Hiking on this remote path, watching my students, I made it a point to jump over rocks and not go around them. That is because my energy was so high I could almost fly. The fact that I was being seen by my students also gave me energy to keep on this path without feeling tired. I was smiling, having a good time, a sense of love and need to share — that was what I could connect with in myself.

*   *   *

As I brought out my image I was definitely aware of a wellspring of energy within me. The exact origin of this energy did not interest me at the time. I simply *rode* the crest of the wave. My "little critic" was mostly kept at bay.

*   *   *

I was aware of a spring of joy flooding through me. I felt wonderfully alive and open and able. There was the presence of music and I felt creative, as if a great reservoir of energy had suddenly been tapped — the faucet opened — and energy poured into my SELF!

* * *

The experience of connecting with and becoming my image was an intense, centered one. I was unaware of my surroundings, and had a sense of timelessness — a suspended time. The image was clear with sharp colors, sounds, and sources. I felt very alive, powerful when I became the image. There was a clear surge of energy which seemed to open up new possibilities. When I returned from this experience, I retained the feeling of optimism and new possibilities. Now, several weeks later, when I recall the experience, I can remember clearly the feeling of aliveness and heightened awareness which accompanied connecting with my energy.

* * *

My energy level was heightened after guided imagery. I don't understand the cognitive processes that lead to increased levels of energy. However, I felt *revitalized*. My image is that of a catalyst for change. Connecting my work to my image reaffirmed for me that I was in the right occupation and that it would bring me many intrinsic rewards for years to come.

* * *

Several participants mentioned that becoming their image was associated with feelings of calmness and peace.

During the most successful periods of guided imagery, I felt a great sense of relief, quiet, and solitude. It was a time of emotional calmness, and at the end of the sessions I felt distinctly relaxed yet at the same time excitingly rejuvenated. This sense of rejuvenation I now see as being a necessary preface to the strong feeling of energy-release which was to follow.

* * *

I seemed to enter "into" myself. I was less aware of those things/people around me; however, I could feel, taste, sense those aspects of my image clearly. No time element! As a choreographer in a dance studio I became part of the film. Felt more relaxed and quiet when I used imagery.

* * *

I was aware of an incredible calm when I became my image. There was an intense feeling associated with my image — actually each of the three times I went through the imagery exercise there were intense feelings. When I experienced my image of teaching and my personal image I felt calm and a sense of satisfaction with my life and teaching. When I connected with my image of wisdom (a Christ-like figure) I felt a sense of hope, joy, and some excitement. Is this connecting with my energy? I know my images were powerful and I wanted to discuss them and I feel good when I recall them.

*   *   *

Yes, I was aware of connecting with my energy. In my image, I was sitting in the chair at the hairdresser's, drinking coffee, listening to music, watching the busy activity around me, a book in my lap, feeling pampered and important, yet relaxed. This feeling was so calming, and that sense of calm was my energy. Then, in my image, I became the hairdresser and I gave that energy, that sense of calm, of being important yet unstressed, to my students, as I tried to accommodate their needs.

*   *   *

Once the connection was made, I immediately felt a sense of well-being, a safe oasis. I felt I was in a world free from constraints and outside influences. I felt refreshed and able to cope in many new ways. I became possessed by my image and found it attached itself to me with vigor. I found myself adding more sensory input to it and the more I added the more energetic I felt. The elasticity of the image caused me to feel very energetic as different scenarios of my image were explored in my mind. As I recalled my image later (many times) I found it soothing!

Other participants responded that the image was valuable, but not necessarily in terms of energy connection:

I believe in the value of imaging but I did not experience a connection with my energy. Perhaps I needed more practice. I found it energy draining. I was probably overly concerned with making my image fit reality. (I know it doesn't have to fit but to be helpful in the future how do you remember what fantasy you created if it isn't reality-based?) Yet I believe imagery is important in communicating complex issues — particularly to visual learners.

*   *   *

As I brought out my image on my own, I was *not conscious* of a connection with my energy. It may have been more of a subconscious connection because I found that: a) I could describe more about my teaching through my image than in reality; b) I was able to present more of a philosophical view of my teaching via the image.

*   *   *

I wouldn't describe it as energy, but more as clarity: a realization of how I see myself as I work and how I regard the people around me and my clients. This was quite useful, and I think will provide me with energy as I return to the situation this fall.

Here are some others:

> Yes, I was constantly aware of connecting to my energy. However, initially this connection was somewhat blurred by: a) my indecisiveness on where I stood in the image, and b) the narrowness of the image itself. Solving these problems made the connection much easier. Knowing where I stood in my image helped me focus my energy. Extending the image gave me the space to release my energy.

*   *   *

> I am not sure what is meant by "connecting with your energy." I know that I had difficulty in becoming my image. I do not think the atmosphere was conducive to letting my imagination go. I think my back problem hindered the process as well. However, I did feel more excitement when I transferred from third to first person process in my descriptions. The image of coach, and what I was trying to accomplish, was clearer in my mind.

One person needed to share in order to connect (the topic of the next chapter):

> As I brought out and became my image, I had a growing awareness of connecting with my energy. In the initial attempt to form my personal image, I experienced some difficulty. I was able to identify an image of my teaching from a positive professional experience. The difficulty arose when I tried to become part of the image. I kept getting "stuck," kept slipping into reality. Working with a partner provided the opportunity to "become" my image. Her questions and clarification techniques allowed me to experience my image much more intensely. My partner helped me to fill in the empty spaces in the "garden" — to see, hear, and smell the activity in the "garden." My image came alive for me and I was aware of connecting with the energy as I became a part of it.

The following emphasizes the sustaining value of their energy:

> I experienced a sense of connecting to my "center" — some place inside me that knows what's right for me. I felt "empowered," not in the sense of now being able to boss people around, but in the sense of having strong hopefulness. I feel I have a place (starting point) to go back to if things get rough.

The documentation for the beneficial effects of evoking and experiencing personal images is compelling. In most cases, it is associated with a direct connection to personal energy. It also connects us with qualities ranging from calmness to clarity which are needed as resources. Chapter Four explores the impact of sharing images on the release of personal energy.

CHAPTER FOUR

Sharing as Co-Creation: Releasing Energy

"Share: To partake of, use, experience, or enjoy with others"

Webster's Dictionary

In this chapter I discuss how sharing personal images serves to release personal energy. My understanding of the power of sharing, portrayed in Figure 5, has evolved gradually from my experience with and observation of student/colleagues. I have also come to realize that we do not experience the release of energy automatically through exchanging words with another person. Releasing energy requires a special kind of transaction and relationship between two persons, a relationship I call *sharing as co-creation.*

Figure 5
The Role of Sharing in Energy Cycles

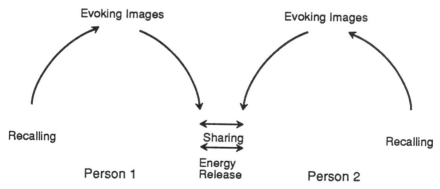

Like the word "image," the word "sharing" has many meanings. Therefore some of you may react negatively to the idea of sharing because your experience of what you have called sharing was less than satisfactory. Again, I invoke your good will and patience as I try to describe the special meaning of sharing as co-creation. It is certainly much more than two people talking with each other or children performing "show and tell." It is a special attitude and tone in the relationship which permits the release of energy: therefore, it is essential to understand, and perhaps experience, this necessary condition.

Initially, I describe sharing as co-creation in the specific situation of two persons sharing their personal images. Later, I consider how the characteristics of sharing as co-creation can enhance interpersonal relationships more generally.

Figure 5 summarizes the process of sharing as it facilitates energy release, thus setting the foundation for transforming energy into action, the subject of the next chapter. This figure highlights how sharing is essential, indeed serves as the flash point, for energy release. Like other concepts I have introduced, sharing as co-creation is not entirely new. For example, it is similar to the "learning partnerships" described by Robinson, Saberton, and Griffin (1985) which also seem to facilitate energy release.

Sharing Images With a Partner

After two people have identified their personal images, they are invited to clarify and elaborate their images through a specific exercise, as follows:

Clarification

1. The first person describes his or her image from inside — the experience of being in the image, feelings, other features, and so on.
2. The partner listens carefully and tries to become a "mirror with feelings," raising questions, non-judgmentally, if this is appropriate. The partner then "plays back" or paraphrases, staying as true to the first person's experience as possible.
3. The first person comments on any new aspects or clarifications arising from the playback as well as his or her feelings about being listened to.

Elaboration

4. The partner enters into the first person's image on his or her own terms, describing all aspects of the experience. At this stage the partner is free to transform and elaborate, and to describe the experience to the first person.

5. The first person considers the elaboration and comments on its effects: new aspects of images, feelings of energy, and so on.
6. The first person and the partner reverse roles and go through the five steps again.

Below is an example, based on the exchange between Sheila (whose image of the rushing stream appeared in Chapter One) and Kit (whose image is found in Appendix 4).

Focusing on Sheila's image

The image is that of a bubbling stream, questing for new directions and places. My stream often meets up with others, and in the ensuing whirlpool we exchange ideas, energy, and support. We progress along together, larger, more powerful, and more content. However, when the other streams leave to pursue their own directions, I experience a feeling of loss. This is where the positive force of imaging came through. I was able to change that feeling. There was a positive sense of the speed and energy of the two or many streams interacting and working together — and a sense of both parties being enriched. Then, when the other left, there was no longer a sense of isolation, but a sense of affirmation, strengthening, rolling along as a river. I have changed — I am enriched, larger, smoother-traveling. In my traveling, I have built in many bays of solitary rest, to regain energy, to relax, to reflect, as well as many whirlpools of interchange. Finally, I must know there is a destination — where and its nature are still unknown, for I must preserve some mystery in my life. But it is there — some place wonderful.

As Sheila describes her experience of being a rushing stream, Kit listens carefully and, where appropriate, asks questions related to the image. Then she "plays back" what she has heard with an emphasis on the feelings Sheila has expressed. Sheila's comments show her reaction:

Clarification.

Working with Kit to reinforce my image was very positive. She helped me focus on surrounding lands and on the feelings I experienced — the eagerness, the openness, the loneliness, and the confident sense of growth ahead.

Elaboration. Kit entered into the image of the rushing stream and found herself experiencing the variety of colors very intensely. Kit's experience helped Sheila to elaborate and extend her original experience of the image:

Kit helped me think in colors while I had focused only on greens, blacks, and whites. I firmed up my image while still managing to retain its original power.

Notice how the listening partner provides the catalyst for the release of energy. In the clarification phase, Kit raises Sheila's awareness of her feelings as well as her inner sense of the image. In the elaboration phase, Kit helps her partner extend the image to other senses and to other aspects. Of course, in the elaboration phase, Sheila need not accept Kit's transformation into her own experience; this is her choice. Now they switch roles.

Focusing on Kit's Image

I see myself as a bright, colorful, transparent bubble that floats above a flock of Canada geese who are making their path toward the small lake. This bubble is alive and radiant with color because I see myself as an outgoing, friendly person. As I float in the air, I pulse in and out: I jump high: I wrap myself around my colleagues (the geese).

As time passes, the bubble bursts forth and starts exploding into millions of bubbles. As the bubble transforms its shape, it jumps higher with energy. It begins to wrap itself around the geese, touching and interacting with the flock. Sensing new confidence, direction, and acceptance, the bubble is now having more fun interacting with the flock. However, the bubble usually knows that it needs time to rest, observe, listen, and reflect, even though the bubble enjoys action almost immediately. The exploration and experimentation continues. There is a sense of "one," sharing new ideas and building positive attitudes.

Clarification. Sheila listens to Kit's description of being in her image, then plays it back as faithfully as possible, with an emphasis on inner feelings. Kit comments:

I liked the idea of sharing images because it gave me more insight into the growth of the image. I felt in unison with my image; I knew where I was journeying. In describing my experience to my partner, I became aware of the panoramic view of the surroundings.

Elaboration. Sheila enters into the bubble image on her own terms, experiences it as liberating, buoyant, and exhilarating.

Again, remember that Kit is not required to elaborate her image based on Sheila's version. She may listen to and respect Sheila's version, and retain her version based on her original experience. Since both parties are actively involved in sharing as co-creation, their success depends on the interpersonal climate as well as their willingness and competence in taking on the attitudes of the other (to be described in more detail later).

At this point, we may consider whose energy is released in the process of sharing. In most cases, the release of energy comes from your own image — for example, Sheila experiences a release of energy as Kit helps her to clarify and elaborate her image of the rushing stream. However, occasionally, the listening partner may experience a surge of energy through entering into the partner's image. As Figure

5 depicts, what occurs is a mutual release of energy. Following are some other comments from students/colleagues after sharing their personal images with a partner:

> I was surprised at how my image unfolded. It allowed me to envision myself in relation to others in my image environment in a non-verbal way. I believe this made a richer and more rewarding experience.

* * *

> Sharing my image with a partner was very powerful. My partner asked questions that brought my image into sharper focus and her paraphrasing of it provided me with even more insight as well as a very positive feeling about myself (to be listened to with that intensity was a very uplifting experience). It was also quite wonderful to have someone share their image with me.

* * *

> Working with a partner was extremely beneficial in clarifying my personal image. In answering my partner's questions, I filled in the details of my own image.

* * *

There is a delicate balance between the value of sharing and the potential negative effects of anticipating "going public." Evoking one's personal image is a private process, as the following candid response illustrates:

> How much do I really want to divulge? How much am I willing to let go? Even my wife reminds me of the walls and barriers which I sometimes erect. I am basically a very private individual, who only comes out of his shell when the situation feels right.

Benefits of Sharing as Co-Creation

Based on the experience of student/colleagues who have engaged in this exercise, there are many benefits.

1. Emotional support

It is revealing about our current culture that we seldom experience someone who listens carefully to our words and feelings. The effect of this "mirror with feelings" is to feel understood and accepted, a seemingly simple yet unfortunately infrequent experience in our interpersonal relations. The loneliness many people feel is certainly not unrelated to their need to be listened to and heard. Such affirmation of our experience is vital to well-being.

2. Promotes confidence

Closely related to feeling emotionally heard is an increase in confidence. This comes through being heard as well as through listening to your partner transform your image. Many experienced practitioners initially feel shaky about the value of their inner wisdom so that working with a colleague who values it is very affirming. Indeed it is the mutual affirmation of co-creation.

3. Increases understanding

Listening to your partner's playback of your thoughts and feelings as well as his or her elaboration of your image often serves to extend and enrich your inner knowledge along new lines. Sometimes, the enrichment occurs through extending your image to other senses, sometimes through new relations and connections within the image.

4. Offers new perspectives

As will be described in the next chapter in detail, the sharing of personal images often shows us new ways of viewing and thinking about situations. Entering into the image of another is often a valuable way of relinquishing an old world view and taking a fresh look at your life and work.

5. Releases energy

Sharing as co-creation is the flash point which ignites energy in both persons who are seeking the basis for the next benefit.

6. Provides a basis for planning action

Sharing personal images is a form of "emotional brainstorming" which provides both the energy and the inner knowledge to plan our actions (see Figure 2).

Characteristics of Sharing as Co-Creation

Sharing as co-creation is characterized by the attitudes of the participants as well as by the tone of their relationship. Before outlining the qualities of this creative process, I invite you to bring out your own implicit notions of a positive relationship by turning to Appendix 5, which provides a variation of the Role Concept Repertory Test. Then you may wish to compare your values with the five qualities of sharing as co-creation discussed below.

I propose that sharing as co-creation involves the following attitudes or qualities on the part of both persons: (1) good will, (2) respect for self and other, including acceptance of the other's wish not to disclose information, (3) a non-judgmental orientation, (4) openness to one another's feelings, and (5) willingness to trust oneself and the other person. These characteristics are based on my experience and observation of student/colleagues sharing and writing together, but as I will discuss in the final section, they may be applied more generally.

1. Good will

Since I have frequently invoked your good will in earlier pages, you know how much I value this quality. It involves a willingness to risk trying something new because of its potential value. "Try it, you may like it" is the stinger invoking good will. No one enters every new situation or meets every new person with uncondi-tional good will; the attitude varies with the situation. It is quite natural to go through a brief review of potential benefits and disadvantages before entering into a relationship, and often there is really very little to lose and considerable to gain. Sometimes, some clarification of the nature of the relationship needs to be negotiated, for example, whether the sharing between the two partners will be private or not, before the good will is extended.

2. Respect

This refers to respecting not only the other as a person with particular views and ideas which may differ from your own, but also the other's right to choose not to disclose or share at a particular time. Sharing as co-creation must be voluntary on both sides, and must be continually open to the choice of both parties to disclose or to keep things private. This seeming contradiction is perhaps the most essential quality of the process, and when sharing is forced, it immediately loses its potential for igniting our energy.

3. Non-judgmental orientation

Just as it is essential in evoking images to suspend critical judgment, so it is with sharing as co-creation. As Figure 5, and more especially Figure 3, depicts, this process is intended to release energy and to allow it to flow freely into our actions. Such free flow is cut off immediately when the Critic appears. A non-critical, accepting atmosphere facilitates the flow of feelings, ideas, and perceptions, while a critical attitude curdles, cuts off, and dries up the flow. Again, note that you are invited to *suspend* critical judgment, not abandon it. As discussed in the next chapter, your critical judgment can be retrieved when you begin to consider your action plans emerging from your energy release through sharing.

4. Openness to feelings

Sharing as co-creation occurs at an emotional as well as an intellectual level, so both parties need to be open to their inner feelings as well as to the emotional barometer of their partner. In relation to Figure 5, the flow of energy in the renewal process takes place primarily in our emotions and feelings, so the process is, in one sense, an opening to our feelings, and an enhancement of this emotional sense through sharing with another. When you consider opening yourself to another in this way, you immediately sense your vulnerability and the necessity for the relationship to be an accepting, non-judgmental one. It must also be one of trust, the final characteristic.

5. Trust

Trust is something which develops over time, so the initial quality is a willingness to trust on the part of both persons. A trusting relationship and how it evolves is not easy to describe. One way of facilitating trust is for the two persons to discuss what each hopes to gain from this transaction. Trust, like good will, is not offered in every situation to every person. Therefore, it may be valuable for partners to negotiate both their mutual intentions and how they might be achieved.

These five qualities form a value orientation to interpersonal relations which can be seen in many diverse areas. At a simple level, one might say that these five qualities define a "good listener," and thus are the goals of training in active listening. At a more comprehensive level, these qualities are often the underlying objectives of professional training in the helping professions such as counseling, social work, teaching, nursing, clinical psychology, and so on. It is assumed in the first instance that one can learn these attitudes in a relatively brief time through listening exercises. In the second instance it is assumed that pre-professional education, which requires several years, will imbue potential professionals with the appropriate attitudes and ideals. Both cases acknowledge that these are ideals to aim for, and that not only do persons vary in terms of their capacity to display each of these qualities, but that individuals vary in displaying these qualities in different situations. (In Chapter Six, I extend the five dimensions of sharing as co-creation into a Spirit of Renewal framework.)

Overcoming Resistance to Sharing as Co-Creation

External obstacles

When two persons participating in sharing as co-creation are in the same organization, their relationship may be hampered by their positions in the organization, and the values the organizational culture places on sharing. For example, if two persons are at *different* levels of the organizational hierarchy, then the power and control which one person holds over the other will likely interfere with developing a constructive relationship, especially in relation to openness and trust. In order for a principal and a teacher to share in this way, the principal must temporarily relinquish his or her power and control.

If two persons are at the *same* level in the organization, this poses a different obstacle, that of potential competition. For example, if the organizational culture is highly competitive, rewarding individual achievement and ideas over mutual productivity and co-operation, then the participants are not likely to be willing to be open, trusting, and non-critical. Therefore, the first requirement is to cultivate the attitudes and relationships which foster trust and creativity within the organizational culture. This is also why it is so difficult to introduce co-operative learning into classrooms which have always operated on a competitive basis.

Internal obstacles

If you transform the dimensions in Table 6 into personal characteristics rather than interpersonal qualities, then you can quickly see that there are variations among people in the attitudes necessary for sharing as co-creation. You may wish to go through these five qualities and form a tentative impression of yourself with respect to each one.

1. How would you characterize yourself in terms of you willingness to try something new as opposed to being wary? (Good will)
2. How strong is your Critic? Do you tend to look for faults and flaws initially? How difficult is it for you to "lighten up" and experience another person or situation? (Non-judgmental orientation)
3. Are you able to detach yourself from your own beliefs and attitudes to listen to different views even though you do not agree with them? (Respect)

4. Are you in touch with your own feelings? Can you sense another person's feelings from what they say and how they act, or is the area of emotions a mystery to you? (Openness to feelings)
5. Are you willing to trust another person initially, or at least discuss the conditions under which you would be willing to explore the possibilities of a trusting relationship? (Trust)

I do not want to leave the impression that our individual variations in willingness to take on these five attitudes is an individual difference which is innate and unchanging. Our attitudes toward sharing tend to come from earlier experiences, and often our resistance or wariness comes not from fixed personality characteristics but from earlier negative experiences in which we have found the effort to share painful or, perhaps in the lesser case, of no value whatsoever.

Just as many people resist personal images because they seem initially to be rather impractical and irrational, so many people feel that sharing is at best a waste of time and at worst a violation of privacy. Such resistance can usually be traced to negative experiences in which the person has (1) taken the risk of disclosing him- or herself to another and has been hurt through becoming vulnerable, (2) participated in sharing with good will but found it had no value, or (3) experienced the other's lack of understanding rather than good will. Whatever the reason in past experience, many people are wary of trying to share again.

A workshop participant may ask, "Why do I have to share to renew myself? Why can't I work with my inner wisdom on my own and achieve the same effect?" My reply is that it may be possible to achieve the benefits of energy release on your own — I cannot say it is impossible — but I have found that I need others to continue on the cycle of renewal, and I have found that, for example this is true for most of the participants in my workshops. Also, sharing as co-creation affords many benefits beyond energy release, and these are very difficult to achieve on your own.

If you are interested to explore, at minimum risk, the phenomenon of sharing, then you might begin gradually. Select a partner whom you already trust and try the exercise on sharing images with a partner. Feel free to discuss your reservations as you go along; feel free to clarify the understanding of the relationship, especially whether what is said will remain confidential and whether you have the choice throughout the exercise to share or retain your ideas and feelings. It is only in a situation of security and low risk that we can begin to share our ideas and feelings.

Characterizing Interpersonal Relations

Table 6 provides a specific tool for applying the ideal qualities discussed in this chapter to two-person transactions. If you have completed the exercise in Appendix

5 you may use your own dimensions; using either your own or those in Table 6 answer the following questions about a specific relationship with another person in you life:

- How close is your relationship to the ideal of sharing as co-creation?
- To what extent would you like it to move toward the ideal?
- Consider how this relationship was in the past.
- How much has it moved in the past and in what direction?

Table 6
Characterizing relationships in terms of their Sharing as Co-creation

Persons in relationship: _____ and _____

Setting of relationship: _____

Characterize this relation by rating on each dimension:

Ideal	Opposite
Good will..	Wariness
Non-judgmental...................................	Critical
High Respect.......................................	Low Respect
Open to feelings..................................	Closed to feelings
High Trust...	Low Trust

Note that you can use this table for planning to improve or modify a relationship. First you might characterize the relationship from your perception and then invite your partner to do the same. After comparing your different views, you might then consider whether you wish to change or develop the relationship in a specific direction, for example, move toward mutual respect. Once a mutually agreed upon goal is established, you can discuss what each of you might specifically do to help you move toward that objective. For example, to increase mutual respect, each person might pay special attention to his or her non-verbal reactions and try to respond in respectful ways. The dimensions in Table 6 provide a blueprint for mapping proposed future movement and development which in turn calls for a plan to bring such movement about. Using the framework in this way brings us closer to the topic of the next chapter, moving into action.

Table 6 provides a framework for portraying the underlying attitudes which inform a relationship between two people. When they want to change the relationship, one or both persons will probably need to consider acquiring or improving specific skills which are related to the general characteristics outlined in the table. Skills in active listening, for example, would include paraphrasing what has been heard, capturing the emotional aspects of what is said, tolerating silence, and so on. For partners to share, they also need the skill of expressing feelings and being open to new perspectives. These skills are often emphasized in professional education, but they may also be the objective of individual learning and development.

The framework in Table 6 and/or the personal framework of interpersonal dimensions brought out in Appendix 5 can serve many practical purposes. For example, when an experienced teacher and a beginning teacher begin working together in an "induction" or "mentoring" relationship, this framework would provide a basis for negotiating their relationship. Both persons would bring out their dimensions and indicate how they would like to work together through characterizing their intentions. They would also continuously monitor the relationship by means of ongoing descriptions. If they found the relationship falling short of their hopes, then their discussion could proceed on what to do about it. As implied earlier, experienced teachers must suspend their hierarchical or informal power over the beginning teacher for this to work. From this example, it should be clear that the framework can be used in many interpersonal situations: supervisor-doctoral student, counselor-client, consultant-client, teacher-student, and so on.

If one or both parties in the relationship is either unwilling to consider it or denies any problem in the relationship, then a different approach is needed, such as counseling. However, when sharing as co-creation operates on these principles, it definitely leads to energy release as described in the next chapter.

CHAPTER FIVE

C-RE-A-T-E: Transforming Energy into Action

"Images and metaphors are not only interpretive constructs or ways of seeing, they also provide frameworks for action. Their use creates insights that often allow us to act in ways that we may not have thought possible before."

Gareth Morgan

This chapter describes the C-RE-A-T-E Cycle, a five-step creative problem-solving approach based on the Kolb Cycle which has been designed to assist participants in transforming energy into action. The acronym comes from the first letter(s) in each step:

1. Concern
2. REflect
3. Action plan
4. Try out
5. Experience

Figure 6 shows these steps in the cycle.

Figure 6
The C-RE-A-T-E Cycle

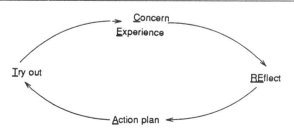

The C-RE-A-T-E Cycle was designed to enable practitioners to develop and apply action plans related to their concerns (Hunt, 1987, pp. 157-160). Yet its success depends on the degree to which participants have brought out their personal images and inner wisdom (Chapter Three) and have been able to work together in a spirit of sharing as co-creation (Chapter Four). These distinctive features need emphasis before further describing the C-RE-A-T-E Cycle.

Prior to working together, participants in the C-RE-A-T-E Cycle need to bring out their experienced knowledge and summarize it on a Resource Sheet (see Table 2). To emphasize this step, I have added two letters to the acronym, RE for Resources, so that it becomes the RE-C-RE-A-T-E Cycle. When I conduct workshops I encourage group members to think of the work of the RE-C-RE-A-T-E Cycle as an opportunity to tap into their inner resources (see Appendix 2) and get them flowing. In a similar way, the Sharing Images With a Partner exercise described in Chapter Four provides a valuable foundation for group members to become more directly aware of the resources available in the group. Specifically, Kit and Sheila might share their personal images with one another, and two other group members in the C-RE-A-T-E group might do the same, before they go through the steps.

The Cycle is illustrated in the first section of this chapter by several examples. Next, I discuss and illustrate each of the five steps in the cycle. Later, I discuss how it might be used with larger groups. The chapter concludes with verbatim comments from participants describing the degree to which they found that sharing released energy and provided the basis for transforming it into action.

Going Through the Cycle: Two Examples

In the following example, Sheila works in a C-RE-A-T-E group with Kit and two other colleagues to address her concern. (Groups usually consist of three or four persons.)

If I were a rushing stream

1. Concern: As a consultant, I work with many teachers of grades 7-12. Many of these teachers are new to teaching and need assistance in planning and management strategies; others have many years of experience and are seeking information and guidance about specific areas. Usually, I react to their calls, and handle each as it comes. While this brings a freshness and individualization to each case, I have begun to sense a lack of freshness on my part. In order to perform more effectively, I would like to set up an action plan to organize my

consulting process, to make it more of a two-way street, and to be proactive where possible.

2.   REflect: I selected the image I have created from among those of the group. While I felt the others had things to offer, mine was the one I was most comfortable with and knowledgeable about. The image is that of a bubbling stream, questing for new directions and places. My stream often meets others, and in the ensuing whirlpool we exchange ideas, energy, and support. We progress along together, larger, more powerful, and more content. However, when the other streams leave to pursue their own directions, I experience a feeling of loss. This is where the positive force of imaging came through. There was a positive sense of the speed and energy of the two or many streams interacting and working together — and a sense of both parties being enriched. Then, when the other left, there was no longer a sense of isolation, but a sense of affirmation, strengthening, rolling along as a river. I have changed — I am enriched, larger, smoother-traveling. In my traveling, I have built in many bays of solitary rest, to regain energy, to relax, to reflect, as well as many whirlpools of interchange. Finally, I must know there is a destination — where and its nature are still unknown, for I must preserve some mystery in my life. But it is there — some place wonderful.

3.   Action plan: I will be open to the directions and motivations of other people (streams). I will take time to get to know them, listen to them, and get their ideas on how to begin to meet their needs. I'll share with them some of my own feelings, give them a sense of where I am in my journey, and encourage them to share and give a sense of where they are in their journeys.

I will enjoy the time of the whirlpool. This is a time for sharing, where each of us will benefit.

There is no loss after a client leaves. Rather there is an enrichment of myself from the interaction. I must hold onto this image and this feeling, because a feeling of disenchantment, of constantly giving and never receiving, could dangerously creep up on me.

4.   Try out: I will build in times of quiet, times when I can reflect, collect my thoughts, plan, and relax, times of independent writing and searching.

On another level, I would like to design a feedback sheet which will help me in the gathering of ideas and information from my clients. One could be for the new teachers I meet in August and could provide me with information about their needs and concerns as well as background and ideas they have to share with others. Another could be a systematization of the process I undergo with each client, providing background information, future needs and actions for me to follow up on, future actions for the client to fall back on, and some kind of a feedback mechanism so that contact is maintained, and I have a sense of the direction of the other person.

Lastly, I must find a way to hold onto this image and its feelings. I know full well that in the maelstrom of the first months, with all the old pressures and new ones, this feeling will be difficult to recapture. I will search for photos — a series of them while up at the cottage next week. I know just where I'll go — it must have been in my subconscious — the headwaters of the lake. I'll place these photos in my office to remind me of the healing, energizing force of my image of streams. [Note that since Sheila evolved her plan during a summer course, she is anticipating its application in the fall.]

5. Experience: Some green lights I hope to see in my clients:
    *   opening up and sharing their experiences with me,
    *   questioning and self-exploration, not just receiving information,
    *   generating excitement and energy,
    *   creating ideas or plans to put into practice, and
    *   positive feelings, a sense of accomplishment, and a balance of input.

In this case, Sheila used her own image, that of a rushing stream, to guide her actions. In the following example, Diana chose to use the image of her colleague, Daphne, to apply to her concern.

If I were clearing the fog

1. Concern: The concern I identified was a desire to communicate more effectively at work, especially in a group setting (e.g., staff meetings). Rather than being able to listen to the concerns raised by others, I find myself feeling threatened. All my energy is focused on me — protecting myself from perceived threats. I wanted to decrease my own defensive behavior and be able to stay tuned to the concerns and issues identified by the group.

2. Reflect: My own image, that of an hourglass, did not seem to provide me with

any new creative energy for dealing with this concern. It seemed flat and static and I was unable to apply it. One of my colleagues, Daphne, shared her image and I immediately felt it could work for me. She described teaching in a room filled with fog. When the students were actively involved in learning, the fog would clear and she could maintain a visual connection with them. When the students were not involved, the fog would thicken and she would be unable to see them, by which time she knew she had lost them. She would try various ways of reconnecting with them. The role became one of clarifying, re-stating, re-framing until she could see her students clearly again.

3. Action plan: Even as Daphne first described this image, I was excited by its possibilities for me. I decided to try it at the next staff meeting two days away. I resisted any in-depth analysis or planning by the group of how I could implement this image. Instinctively, I felt I could use it without any concrete plan of action. In fact, I felt that trying to focus critical thinking or problem-solving skills on the situation was counter-productive at this time. The beauty of the image for me was its simplicity. I would simply live it.

4. Try out: At the next staff meeting I tried it out. I attempted to see each group member clearly at all times and to focus on what they were saying. When a comment was made that provoked my defensiveness I could see the group fade away — the fog moved in. Rather than allowing my attention to focus on myself (in perceived self-protection) I worked at focusing on the group members, clearing the fog, and really hearing what was being said. Many times during that meeting the fog moved in and was dissipated again. I had to suspend my critical thinking/judgment and just go with the image. It felt fairly comfortable to do this. I was surprised at how well it worked and how much more I learned about the workplace conflicts.

5. Experience: The problem has not been solved but I know that if I can eliminate the barrier of my defensiveness I will be able to engage in the kind of communication that is essential for problem solving.

    Daphne's reaction to Diane's using her image follows:

    > I was delighted when a classmate utilized my image to help her solve a problem she was having. She reported significant improvements in her comfort level as a result.

    There are a number of differences in the two examples which are important. In

Sheila's case, the wisdom of the image is used to develop an explicit plan of action. In Diane's case, critical judgment is suspended so that she can "go with the image" which then guides her actions. Depending on the nature of the concern and the person using the image, one or the other may prove appropriate, as we will see in later examples. In both cases, the image provides the necessary new perspective.

How to Use the C-RE-A-T-E Cycle

There is a certain irony in giving specific steps and instructions for creative problem-solving because the process must be free and spontaneous if it is to work. I usually introduce my instructions with the suggestion that they provide a structure for creativity. If time permits, I encourage colleagues to work in pairs, sharing as described in the last chapter, to develop a sense of the essential qualities: good will, non-judgmental orientation, respect, openness, and trust.

To demystify creative group work, I often introduce the C-RE-A-T-E Cycle by indicating that it is a tool to open up the resources of the group and to allow these resources to flow so that they can be applied to specific concerns. I also note that one of the reasons personal images are valuable in creative problem-solving is that they provide a new way of thinking about our concerns. To state our concerns is to acknowledge that we are stuck, and images often help us become "unstuck." The following sections elaborate the specific steps of the cycle in detail.

Step 1: Identify Your Concern

Group members receive a C-RE-A-T-E sheet (Appendix 6) on which to write their concerns. They are asked to take account of three criteria, namely that their concern is (1) applicable to *professional* issues (although C-RE-A-T-E may be applied to personal/domestic concerns), (2) stated as *specifically* as possible in relation to another person or a specific topic or assignment, and (3) within an area for which responsibility can be taken.

I usually suggest some areas from which concerns might be selected: (1) communicating more effectively, (2) initiating some change in practice (e.g., learning a new approach), (3) initiating some specific self-change or development (e.g., developing the capacity for being more open to feelings), and (4) initiating some form of professional renewal or improvement in organizational climate.

Improving communication. The concern needs to be stated specifically, for example:

> I would like to communicate more effectively and get along better with the teacher with whom I will work next year.

> I would like to communicate better with a colleague with whom I am compelled
> to work. I find her very dominating.

The process of stating a concern more specifically is familiar to counselors and consultants who spend considerable time helping their clients state their concerns in a form which can be dealt with. In the C-RE-A-T-E Cycle, as in counseling and consultation, the concern needs to be clarified and directly related to the person expressing the concern so that a practical plan of action can be developed. Concerns stated ambiguously and generally cannot be constructively addressed; neither can those which involve another person's making the change. They must involve the person directly and specifically.

Change in practice. Two examples follow:

> My concern is that the environment within my classroom may be too structured.
> I may not be providing a consistent opportunity for children to assume an active
> role in their own learning. I see myself now as "imparter of knowledge" as
> opposed to "facilitator of learning."

> I am going back to teaching after being at home with my children for seven
> years. At this point I would like to alter my "mode" of teaching. This exercise
> has provided me with the opportunity to examine how I might bring about this
> change.

Self change. This area is, of course, closely related to change in practice:

> How to become more sensitive to, and how to best address, students' individual
> needs, in the context of a trade school (secondary level) with a population of 200
> low-ability students.

The following example is not only specific, but indicates some green lights:

> In the coming months I will be faced with the task of presenting myself in
> interviews because I am seeking a more challenging position. I often feel less
> than adequate in these situations and I realize that I do not always interpret
> questions "correctly," nor do I relax sufficiently to allow my real strengths and
> talents to emerge.
> I want to attend interviews in a relaxed, yet confident state. I want to
> understand the questions and respond to them in a clear, concise, and compre-
> hensive fashion. Above all, I want to project a sense of confidence in my ability
> to deal with challenges.
> I know I would be successful if I could be aware of the interview team, if I
> could read their faces and bodies as well as their voices and their words. I would
> be successful if, in my center, I felt CALM and could send out the previously
> mentioned warm light to them, *through* me.

The next example shows how group members can help clarify a concern:

> I expressed my concern to the class as well as to my C-RE-A-T-E group. I had difficulty expressing my concern because it seemed to be an undefined feeling of discontent with my work situation. I am concerned by what I view as a lack of caring about students by my organization, and by its callous treatment of many teachers
>
> I initially expressed my concern as "making a major change in my career." I feel that because I cannot change the organization, I'll have to change myself, or leave the organization. Of course this concern was not clearly expressed.
>
> After sharing concerns with my two partners, I clarified my concern as involving changing my approach to the things that distress me at school.

Sometimes, the identified concern is to develop an underdeveloped quality, for example, a Southerner might choose to develop openness to feelings, or as one colleague put it, "Go North, Young Man." (See suggestions for moving along on your journey in Chapter Eight.)

Program initiation. The example below illustrates the specificity of this concern:

> In my role in an intermediate school setting, I am responsible for seeing that suitable programs are in place for adolescent youngsters identified as exceptional and who therefore require individual programming. This means that adaptations must be made to current programs. Part of my function is also to serve as an in-school consultant and provide strategies and whatever support a teacher may need to implement these individualized programs.
>
> In September I will be the co-ordinator of special education for our board and I am concerned about implementing our board policy on integration. There are some teachers who are planning effective integration experiences for their students in self-contained classes, while there are others who are not providing any integration, or poorly planned integration which results in students feeling unsuccessful.

Because of my emphasis on professional renewal, some participants choose to address the concern of planning a professional renewal program for their organization. The following illustrates a concern stated in these terms:

> I was concerned about the negativity expressed covertly and overtly toward my "gifted" students both by staff and members of the student body. I wanted to work toward changing their perception and in so doing lessen the pain that children who are exposed to negativity on a daily basis begin to feel.

This concern might be re-stated by beginning, "What can I do to . . ." or "How can I help. . . ." Concerns need to be expressed in personal terms and include an "I" statement.

After group members have identified their concerns, they read them aloud, and the group chooses one to focus on. When time permits, each concern will be dealt with. Even though there may be similarities in concerns between group members (e.g., two may wish to address communication concerns), the focus should be on the specific concern of one person. Later, implications for others can be considered. Once the specific concern has been identified, it is helpful for the group to emphasize that for the next period of time they will rely only on personal images to deal with this concern: they will not give advice on how to deal with it. (After completing the steps in the cycle, direct advice may be offered.)

Step 2: Reflect and Select an Image

The group member whose concern has been selected is responsible for choosing an image from the images of the other members of the group. This process of choosing an image is a vital step, but it is often not an easy one. When we enter this stage, we are leaving the world of reality where the concern has us stuck and we are entering the world of imagery and fantasy. In the same way that we cannot logically evoke an appropriate personal image, so we cannot logically derive the "right" image for our concern; it is a matter of feeling that it may be right and trying it out — for example, in Diane's case, trying out her colleague's image of a fog lifting. We need to enter into an image to appreciate its essence, then begin, gradually, to apply it to the initial concern by asking such questions as "Where am I in the image?" "Where are the other people?" "How are we related?" Sometimes an image may be full of energy, but it is not appropriate for our specific concern.

The enigma in choosing is that when we first try an image we do not know what new perspectives it will provide. If we knew the new perspectives, we would not need the image. So there is a process of trusting the image, becoming it, and proceeding with the sense that it may prove beneficial in ways we do not know about. This is part of sharing as co-creation, especially the willingness to suspend critical judgment and allow the resources and images to flow freely.

Patience and openness to surprise are essential at this step, and other group members can assist by encouraging the person who is trying out images to enter into them fully before considering their potential value. Notice that it is important to consider positive images that have already been identified and to try not to concoct negative images that portray the concern itself (e.g., a puppet or a prisoner). Negative images simply re-state the concern — and being stuck — at the imagery level.

In the following example, the group member's concern is whether or not to promote another staff member. She responds below, by way of her experience and her own imagery, to each of the images provided by the other group members.

Image I: My work is like a bird that rides the wind, sometimes soaring effortlessly, at other times being buffeted and having to struggle.

> *Rather than using the image of a bird, we thought we would use a kite on a string. The employee would be the kite on a string and I would be controlling*

the kite string. I had the option of keeping the kite string taut and letting it out gradually as the employee was able to take on new challenges or letting it out and watching the kite soar and struggle and grow on its own.

Image II: My work is like a walk down a lonely street amid falling snow.

We tried to work with this image but it didn't seem to be the right fit. The only association we could make was that I was feeling isolated and perplexed about my concern. If I touched one of the falling snowflakes, it might melt . . . whatever decision I made would be a delicate one.

Image III: My work is like a garden.

We related this image in such a way that I was the gardener and the employee was one of the flowers. I was in control of how much water the garden received, how close together the flowers were and how much sun they had. Some flowers needed more care than others. In other words, I was in control of their growth and development. The problem was that I didn't know how much care was needed.

Although this image was closer to my situation, it didn't seem as good as the kite on a string.

Image IV: My work is like a Lego set. Pieces that fit together properly will be formed into a great creation, but if there is a bad fit, the creation will crumble.

After considerable discussion, we selected the "Kite on a String" image. First, the kite is flying, but turbulence is occurring. The type of kite may not be suitable for strong winds. I am holding the kite string and trying to make the kite aerodynamic. Wind, snow, rain are extraneous factors.

Occasionally none of the images offered by the group are appropriate, and in such cases it is perfectly acceptable to consider other images such as those listed in Appendix 4. I have found great variation in participants' willingness to use the images of others. For those who prefer to work with their own imagery, it is sometimes helpful to transform an image by asking it what it needs. For example, one colleague was working unsuccessfully with an image of being a mountain climber. She discovered that she also needed a magic potion to help the climbers complete their climb. Whether you transform your own image or seek images from others or choose them from those listed by others, the key is to be open to the image so that you can fully appreciate and receive its energy.

Personal images are often associated with certain qualities, for example, the quality of gentleness in a humming bird. It also happens that we find an image appropriate because it contains a quality that we need in order to deal with a concern even though we may be unaware of this. For example, Diane's choice of the clearing fog eventually provided her with the qualities of clarity and self-confidence which she needed in her work.

When the C-RE-A-T-E Cycle goes well, there is a free flow of comments and of feelings, something like emotional brain storming, so that when the group member is choosing images and trying them on for size (e.g., "If I were a spider building a web ...") the others help by stretching the image, asking questions, free-associating about how it might be transformed, and so on. This is the secret ingredient of the C-RE-A-T-E Cycle.

Step 3: Action plan

In this step, the person enters into the image gradually, expressing the various parts of the concern with special emphasis on retaining its essential feeling and the relationship between its parts. This is a delicate step, fostered by the other members of the group. The purpose is to open yourself to the wisdom of the image, its qualities, and the relations among the parts. Very gradually, then, the wisdom of the image is transformed into the wisdom of action. Remember that this step may occur in the development of a plan of action, as in Sheila's case, or it may involve trusting the image and entering into it "in the moment" as with Diane. Following is an extended example of the C-RE-A-T-E Cycle up to and including the Try Out stage:

If I Were a Voice Coach

1. Concern: Next September, I will be the Assistant Head of Mathematics at a high school. In June I met my colleagues in the department. I perceived one of them to be resistant to new ideas and to be overly confident that his ways are the best ways. Many of his ideas are good, but he is very young and has only two years of teaching experience. My concern is this: How can I relate to Mr. X in such a way that I can capitalize on his strengths and at the same time encourage him to be more flexible and accepting of other ideas?

2. Reflect: I examined the images of my colleagues in my C-RE-A-T-E Cycle group but none of them seemed quite appropriate. However, from one of the images another emerged: that of a voice coach training a singer for a part in a quartet. In a quartet, each voice has its own characteristics, but the voices must blend to ensure harmony and rhythm. The voice coach, herself a trained singer, also makes suggestions to the lead who sings the melody on how to improve his performance (e.g., projecting his voice, breathing exercises, voice exercises for extending his range, exercises and suggestions for improving tone quality). The voice coach demonstrates all of these things to explain her meaning.

3. Action plan: Applying this image to my concern gave me some ideas on developing a plan of action:

- encourage and provide opportunities for Math Department members to share ideas;
- offer assistance in the implementation of ideas;
- implement some of Mr. X's ideas into my own classroom; and
- show Mr. X the results of some of my own ideas (or those of other colleagues).

4.   Try Out: After a period of time I would expect to see some signs that Mr. X was responding to my plan. I would look for:

- responses such as "I'll give it a try" when I or one of my colleagues suggests, "This seems to work well for me. Have you ever thought of using it?";
- confirmation that Mr. X has gone to other practitioners for suggestions when he has experienced difficulties rather than struggling alone; and
- evidence that Mr. X has actually incorporated into his classroom practice a curriculum/management tool suggested by myself or another colleague.

I most certainly do not want to squelch Mr. X's enthusiasm, but, like a voice coach, I want to bring him into harmony with the others as well as improve his solo ability so that he adds to rather than detracts from the whole.

I also recommend that in developing an action plan you try to identify a few "green lights" which will signal to you that you are on the right track. For example, in trying to communicate better with another person, a green light might simply be that the person takes more notice of you than of others, or perhaps talks more extensively with you than with others. Green lights are not always completely positive, but they flow from the overall action plan to inform us of whether or not we are moving in the right direction. It often takes some time to accomplish a specific intention (i.e., facilitating communication) so green lights help sustain us in the process.

Sometimes it may prove valuable to invite the person about whom you are concerned to enter into the image with us. For example, one group member thought of herself as a bee keeper in considering her role as librarian/resource person in that she was providing the setting for the bees (students) to make their honey (integrate their reports) after they had brought in the pollen (knowledge) from the outlying fields (classrooms). She planned to share this image with classroom teachers as a means of facilitating their joint effort with the students.

Steps 4 and 5: Try Out and Experience

Putting the plan into action and receiving feedback are the last steps in the model. However, remember that this is a cycle and that you may want to reframe and adapt your action plan once you have proceeded through the cycle and have received feedback from the Experience stage.

The following example from Alan shows how the C-RE-A-T-E Cycle plays out over a period of time inside and outside the class/workshop.

I was quite fortunate to be teaching a course while I was taking the Learning Styles course. This allowed me to reflect upon specific events during my teaching and upon students that had definite immediacy. This was particularly useful during our class's work on the C-RE-A-T-E Cycle.

As a result of a guided imagery exercise my image changed from that of a lens, where the light of the student was focused by me, the lens, to that of a prism. In the prism image, the students were still the light, but now as they passed through me, that is, interacted with me, they "changed" into a wide spectrum of colors rather than a thin beam of light. Also, depending upon the orientation of the prism (me) to the light (the students), the light could be reflected away or refracted into a spectrum. I interpreted these aspects of the image to relate to the different personalities of the students, their motivation to learn, my changing personality, and my motivation to teach, any combination of which would result in reflection ("no" learning) or refraction (learning).

In order to experience the C-RE-A-T-E Cycle, the class divided into groups of three with each person identifying "a person with whom you do not communicate as well as you would like." Each person shared their "communication concern" and a decision was made as to which "problem" would become the subject for the C-RE-A-T-E Cycle exercise. As it turned out, we began to use my prism image which evolved into many prisms, similar to a chandelier. In this image both teachers and students were prisms, the light represented learning experiences and depending upon the position of each prism relative to one another the light would be refracted into a colorful pattern or it would be reflected.

It was near the end of the semester, and some of my colleagues were expressing concern about final examinations. Most felt that a final exam was unnecessary, and I agreed. Yet, ironically, before we would meet again I would have given a final exam to my own students! What hypocrisy!

Before I continue, I think that I should describe the situation with the person I had chosen "with whom I did not communicate as well as I would like." She was enrolled in the course I was teaching. (I will call her Jane.) Jane had done very well on a number of assignments for the course. However, the day following the mid-term examination, she telephoned me saying that she had done so poorly on the mid-term that she had received permission to drop the course and would be right over to have me sign the forms. I had not yet marked her exam, and when she arrived we sat down together and I marked the exam with her. Before looking at her written answers, I asked her to answer the questions verbally. She did quite well, certainly much better than on the examination. Further discussion revealed that during the examination she was extremely nervous and wasn't able to focus on the answers to the questions . . . she really hadn't understood the questions. She was particularly stressed because she was on academic probation and needed a C in this and another two courses to remain within the university. I suggested that she take the examination away and rewrite it and I would mark the rewrite and amalgamate the two marks. She seemed relieved and decided not to drop the course.

I was feeling rather concerned about the whole idea of examinations, and since I had some time I drove down to the Beach area of Toronto where I could sit and watch the lake. The sound of the waves lapping at the shore and the gulls overhead helped me relax. I began thinking about examinations: the hypocrisy of my giving a final exam on the one hand and saying that they weren't necessary on the other. I thought about why I felt an examination was necessary in my course, that this had to do with "the fact that it was a science course," and that "good science requires stringent and rigorous evaluation!" I thought to myself. Yet Jane had demonstrated a good grasp of the material and had employed the concepts very effectively. She just couldn't "perform" in a written test situation. "But that's her problem . . . she needs to learn how to be calm during an examination," I thought. "Besides, what would my teaching colleagues think about the quality of *my* course if I didn't have a written final?" The gulls wheeled above me and the waves continued to lap at the shore, and as I watched the sunlight dance off the rippled surface of the water the prism image came back to me. We often expect others to change and yet are not willing to consider any change in ourselves. In the chandelier, both prisms can change, thereby enhancing the quality of the refracted light.

"What if . . . ," I thought, "What if I write up an examination, calculate the mark that each student had based on their term work, calculate that mark out of 100 and tell the students that if they wished to raise that mark they had the option of writing the final, that, however, if they were satisfied with their mark they could opt out of the final?" That's what I did. The C-RE-A-T-E Cycle had helped me solve my problem. As I reflect upon the experience, there are a number of elements which occurred that I think helped in the process:

• having an image;
• sharing my image with two other colleagues;
• reworking my image to help with another's concern;
• hearing about my colleagues' dislike of exams.

Variations on the C-RE-A-T-E Cycle

The C-RE-A-T-E Cycle can be extended beyond the approach described above. The group can be enlarged, the focus can be on a common concern, and/or the group can collectively apply the same image. Note that in the following examples that before the large group variation, members of the large group have previously worked in small groups for it is in small group interaction that energy is released.

Enlarging the group

If we consider a group of 30 participants who have been working in 10 C-RE-A-T-E groups, they can work as a large group in which all of the resources of the total group are directed to the concern of a single group member. This is an extreme example of opening the resources of the group to deal with a concern.

Addressing a common concern

In cases where all group members come from the same organization, it may be appropriate to begin by finding a common concern which they wish to address. This concern may be addressed in small groups and then shared in the total group. This approach is also effective when group members have similar roles — for example, school principals might wish to address a common concern to communicate more effectively with parents.

Applying a common image

All members may be invited to adopt a common image (e.g., "If I were a rushing stream...") which may be applied to individual or common concerns. In either case, opportunity should be allowed to share different variations on the common image so that each may consider further elaboration.

Whatever the variation, the key to success is to maintain a spirit of respect for each other and a belief that such a process may lead to valuable results for all. Of equal importance is that it should be fun. A general rule to keep in mind when applying the C-RE-A-T-E Cycle is that even though the process may be demanding and challenging, it should be enjoyable. If it ceases to be fun, stop and begin again.

Finally, note that although my emphasis is on imagery, you might benefit by exchanging other forms of experienced knowledge, such as stingers, to develop new perspectives from which to derive action plans.

Do Sharing and Applying Images Release Your Energy?

The excerpts below document (1) the relation between sharing images and energy release (Chapter Four) and (2) the relation between applying images and transforming energy into action (this chapter). These responses were made by student colleagues (anonymously) after completing their work with the C-RE-A-T-E Cycle.

> As I began to develop my own image, that of cultivator, and more especially as we began to apply this to professional concerns, both my level of energy and my excitement increased considerably. The C-RE-A-T-E Cycle, in tandem with my personal image, was a very compelling part of the course for me. The process of bringing theory and practice together was energizing.
>
> The group work during these sessions was super. In sharing images and concerns, I discovered a whole new approach which helped me uncover hitherto dormant qualities. As we worked together, I found that I was viewing

issues from perspectives that were new and fresh. This process not only unearthed new perspectives to issues but gave me some very exciting personal insights into my own resources and capabilities. The process of releasing new perspectives and approaches is ultimately energizing. It also speaks eloquently to the wisdom of allowing people to work in groups.

These comments and those that follow came in response to my question,

As you shared your image with your partner and your group, did you experience a release of energy? If so, describe your experience as specifically as possible. If not, what was your experience?

Almost all student/colleagues reported a release of energy in sharing, confirming the assumption that I had made about personal images, sharing, and energy release:

The image which I created on my own generated energy. However, when I shared this image with my partner, the energy doubled and it was amazing how the process of devising an image could be shared, developed, and elaborated with another colleague. To share this, and to convey my excitement and energy with others, was a real source of affirmation. I also felt great about being able to share my colleague's very unique and individual image.

*   *   *

Sharing my partner's image allowed me to see the possibilities of my own image. We were different and yet the same, which gave me a sense of affirmation and support which, in turn, gave me energy to act.

*   *   *

I felt a release of energy which I had not experienced when developing the image on my own. It felt like a "take off." I developed aspects of the image and saw possibilities that I could not have imagined on my own.

*   *   *

I experienced a sense of excitement as I retold my image to the group. It was not so much energy as it was anticipation, a sense of joy and power.

*   *   *

With brainstorming and the supportiveness of the group, action came easily. I felt vital and enthusiastic, as if no problem was unsolvable. (Bring on the next one!)

*   *   *

I felt energy in the group as we shared our images and tried to be the other's image. I felt warmth and acceptance in the group. It was a comfortable and positive atmosphere. The energy grew especially when we did not think that a particular image suited our purpose. Our beliefs came out when we shared our images and concerns. At first the process was slow, but when we got into the images and concerns, energy started to flow because we were sharing ideas. We were trying to give more meaning to the experience.

Following are a few instances in which energy release was not experienced through sharing:

No, I did not experience a release of energy through sharing but from the experience itself. In analyzing it and getting my partner into it I came to some insights and once I caught the insight, I felt the release of a lot of energy. I even needed a few moments to be quiet, to write down what I had learned, and *to do nothing* for a while.

* * *

I do not think I felt a release of energy unless the solving of my concern through imagery may be considered a release of energy. No doubt an amount of energy was released as my colleague and I dialogued, read each other's signals, and flexed our approaches. At any rate I always "feel good" or experience a release of energy whenever there has been transactional contact with another human being.

One person described an alternative experience as follows:

Although there was some energy release, I felt rather relieved and peaceful as a result of my sharing. There was a certain "Ah ha" feeling — so that's it.

Several persons observed that the creative process itself left them drained although they had tapped new sources of energy within themselves:

When we finished each session I was exhausted — completely drained, though I hadn't left my seat. There seemed to be no end to the ideas that we could come up with. When we seemed depleted, someone else could start us all up again with a new direction!

* * *

My release of energy must have been quite complete because I would leave class emotionally drained, although with a great sense of pride in our accomplishments.

* * *

Yes, I would say that I did experience a release of energy when sharing images with a partner. As more and more ideas were expressed, I became more deeply involved in the image. The image expanded in scope and I became exhilarated with all the possibilities. When we finished, we all expressed a feeling of being drained of energy. However, when we worked on the next image we seemed to have developed some stamina.

* * *

I'd call the experience: *draining, intensive, exciting, interesting, and pleasurable.*

Almost all participants experienced energy release by sharing their image with others. There was considerable variation in their response to "living in" another's image. Some, for example, did not experience energy release through experiencing their partner's image:

I could see the image but I had difficulty becoming it and when I did I had some feelings but these came nowhere near the exhilaration I felt when I shared my own image — I think that did release energy since I wrote a poem after sharing my image. Actually the poem took only a minute or two and I hardly remember writing it.

* * *

I felt a greater release of energy when I was sharing my own image than when I was sharing my images with my colleagues. I put my energy into forming the image they were describing and forming questions to help them describe/develop their images.

In other cases, becoming the image of another was quite energizing:

The sharing was a very active and dynamic process. The more information shared, the more we were willing to disclose. Being the other's image allowed me to discover more about myself. I was able to step outside my own parameters and look at myself and my practice through the perceptions of others.

* * *

The experience of sharing and entering into the image of my partner was one of intense connectedness. We were very focused on each other. There was a sense of timelessness, of the lack of surroundings. I was eager to share my image and I responded to my partner's receptivity. Her ability to reflect my image back to me confirmed me and was comforting. When I entered my partner's image, I felt very connected to her. But rather than the intense, exhilarating feelings which I experienced when I entered my own image, I felt detached, peaceful, and rewarded in that she confirmed my description of the feelings within the image. The energy released through the sharing of images seems to be channelled between the partners, bringing about a sense of connection.

Some persons were explicitly aware of energizing others:

> I felt as though I were releasing a sense of calm and that others were receiving it.

Some described having to overcome a resistance before experiencing energy release:

> I found myself resisting the other's image. I did not want the nurturing stance which my partner's image seemed to demand of me. I resisted nurturing others. When I allowed myself to become the image, I began to nurture myself — there was great peace and a feeling of well-being.

Some used another image to describe their energy release:

> Prior to solving the two problems, I felt like steam trying to force the lid off. Luckily, somebody (my colleagues) took the lid off, and the steam (energy) was released. Once the major barrier was eliminated, the steam flowed freely and constantly.

*   *   *

> I had an experience of being charged with electricity. The best way to describe it is to imagine electricity jumping the gap between our two bodies. After class, I felt supercharged, alive, and motivated.

*   *   *

> The sharing did cause a release of energy and a sense of satisfaction also. It was much like "living a good book" and all the ups and downs of the plot and then the smug satisfaction one feels when the book has ended and the characters' problems are at rest.

Sheila's comments conclude this chapter:

> I was able to gain a sense of enrichment and fulfillment after parting with colleagues. I had changed — physically my stream was now a river, fuller, larger, rolling along. Mentally, I was calmer, soothed, enriched by the ideas and memories. The energy released has a power to transform actions and sustain feelings, even in a time of crisis.

CHAPTER SIX

The Spirit of Renewal

"Spirit: Intent, real meaning or characteristic quality"
Webster's Dictionary

This chapter introduces the Spirit of Renewal, a framework of beliefs, images, and qualities which form the core of this book. This framework, however, was not originally a part of my plan; it came as a surprise. I like to think that it came about through my trusting the process of renewal in myself. For it was after sharing the first five draft chapters with my student/colleagues that I came to realize it was time to bring my ideas about renewal into a more comprehensive definition so that they might be applied not only to professional development but also to other areas: organizational support, research, program initiation, pre-professional education, and so on.

The Spirit of Renewal framework in Table 7 exemplifies how trusting in the continuous cycle of renewal and following it with fidelity can lead to unexpected, surprising, and very valuable results. After describing the framework, I discuss how it can be embraced in our personal and professional lives. The Spirit of Renewal framework is illustrated in pre-professional education, the renewing organization and school-based improvement.

Capturing the Spirit of Renewal

The framework portraying the Spirit of Renewal evolved gradually as I wrote, shared draft chapters with colleagues, and reflected on their feedback and comments. It evolved from my early depiction of renewal in Chapter Two as (1) beginning "in here," (2) needing to be shared, and (3) being ongoing. Further evolution occurred as I developed the characteristics of sharing as co-creation, described in Chapter Four as (1) having good will, (2) being non-judgmental, (3) having respect, (4) showing openness, and (5) being trusting. These qualities are also present in the framework.

In bringing out my beliefs, I assumed that beginning with myself was an idea so central to my work that I did not need to express it as a belief. It was the process by which I arrived at my beliefs — the equity of expertise, the synergy of sharing, positive emphasis, and continuity. Once I identified the four beliefs, I was able to evoke my personal images for each one (for example, I associated continuity with traveling on a journey).

In the previous chapter, I touched on the importance of the relation between our personal images and their underlying qualities — for example, a rushing stream may be associated with the quality of freshness or vigor. The underlying quality refers to our personal experience of a particular image, and the related quality may vary from person to person for the same image. The personal images that we use in the C-RE-A-T-E Cycle hold value partly because they provide the quality we need to deal with a concern. Therefore, it seemed important to identify the quality I associated with these beliefs/images (summarized in the right-hand column of Table 7).

When I first reflected on these four qualities — respect, openness, optimism, and patience — I was amazed because I found that I had re-created the qualities to which I personally aspire, even though I had not intentionally set out to do so. There was, however, a quality missing which I value very much, and that was a sense of humor. Maintaining a sense of humor has many meanings — retaining a sense of childlike playfulness, laughing at oneself, enjoying the imperfections of life, and consequently reducing our sense of being stressed. This quality — sense of humor — needed a value/belief, and I came up with contradiction to represent the sense of surprise essential to humor. Contradiction complements continuity nicely, and reminds us of the realities and imperfections on life's journey. Still, I probably would never have identified contradiction as a value had it not been for my wish to include a sense of humor. Finally, there is the overarching belief in human potential, my own and that of others. This central value is the foundation for all the others, and its related quality is faith.

The personal credo expressed as the Spirit of Renewal framework has developed over my lifetime. Earlier, I had tried expressing my values in the context of the principles underlying mutual adaptation (Hunt, 1987, p. 131), but when I developed the Spirit of Renewal framework I felt an exhilarating sense of wholeness because I was able to express my inner beliefs and feelings so clearly. Realizing the very personal significance of this framework, I considered if others might be able to transform it into a personally meaningful guide for themselves. I also considered

Table 7

The Spirit of Renewal: A framework of values, images, and qualities

Value/belief	Personal image	Quality
1. Equity of expertise	Balanced scales; "side by side"	Respect
2. Synergy of sharing	Musicians improvising and "trading fours"	Openness
3. Positive emphasis	Rainbow, Silver lining	Optimism
4. Continuity	Journey	Patience
5. Contradiction	Balloon pops	Humor/Surprise
Overall: Human potential	Cocoon to butterfly	Faith

what meaning my basic beliefs might have for others and how others might gain from my experience. I invited students/colleagues to evoke their own personal images so that the beliefs would take on greater personal meaning. Table 8 summarizes a few of their images.

Table 8
Enriching the Spirit of Renewal with New Images

Value/Belief	Images
Equity of expertise	Snowflakes, each unique, falling to the ground See-saw
Synergy of sharing	Chamber musicians playing "really tight" Making love Horticulturalists sharing gardening tips
Positive emphasis	Sunrise A field of beautiful sunflowers A contented smile
Continuity	A spiral that never ends Salmon swimming to spawn Writing your story
Contradiction	Jack-in-the-box A musical note out of place

In other words, each of us can develop our own Spirit of Renewal framework. In addition to the variation in images, there will be variation in the qualities associated with them. For example, rather than associating the image of the journey with patience, as I did, one student/colleague associated it with surprise. Then there is the issue of whether you might generate your own values/beliefs. One of my colleagues at the University of Toronto's Faculty of Education, Mary Beattie, uses the framework with her pre-service education students, encouraging them to evolve their own personal credos. (This exercise is extremely valuable, though it may not constitute a Spirit of Renewal.)

I invite you to play variations on the framework in Table 7, with your own images and qualities, and then later if you wish to try your hand at expressing your own fundamental beliefs in your own framework, making it your own.

Clarifying the Framework

1. Equity of expertise

I expressed this belief earlier through stingers such as "Every person is a psychologist" and "Experts are persons, too" which are based on my conviction that as participants in the human venture we each develop inner wisdom. To accept the equity of expertise does not mean that every person knows everything or that every person's experienced knowledge is true. It does mean that experienced knowledge in human affairs comes primarily from experience in human affairs, and this applies to ourselves and to others.

Focusing on ourselves, we are likely to regain some confidence when we embrace the equity of expertise. We come to realize that our experience in human affairs is a valid source of knowledge. Focusing on self-proclaimed experts in human affairs we bring out our Critic who asks them, "How do you know that?" and "Show me in your actions." Raising such questions does not show disrespect; rather it is an invitation to the "expert" to address human affairs from the position of those who are participants, not aloof, detached observers (elaborated in Chapter Eight).

My most indelible experiences affirming this belief have occurred while working with student/colleagues in class as we have mutually explored and tried to understand renewal. I learned so much from them that the stinger "Teaching is learning; learning is teaching" took on a powerful meaning for me. We had truly become learners together — equity of expertise in action.

My images for this belief all involve a horizontal equality between persons, not a top-down hierarchical structure — for example, balanced scales, "side by side," or fence posts of equal height holding up a fence. They involve an underlying respect for the other, and more specially, a willingness and capacity to listen in a non-judgmental way to the other's ideas.

2. Synergy of sharing

As we saw above, the equity of expertise does not mean that everyone knows everything; similarly, the synergy of sharing does not require making oneself open and baring one's soul to everyone. To embrace the synergy of sharing, to open oneself to others, is to become vulnerable. Therefore, the synergy of sharing prospers when the nature of the openness has been clarified: open to whom and under what conditions? As noted in Chapter Four, sharing as co-creation requires not only openness, but also respect for the other, and this respect extends to accepting the other's wish not to share at a specific time or to share with some conditions clarified.

As shown in Figures 3 and 4 (pp. 35, 36) the openness in sharing is both an openness to self and openness to the other, or, put another way, an openness to listen and an openness to speak. The more open the participants, the more the energy flows. My images of the synergy of sharing involve creative transformations, such as building and transforming in the spontaneous improvisational exchanges of jazz musicians interweaving their variations on the musical theme.

3. Positive emphasis

"Accentuate the positive" may seem trite until you take it seriously and apply it consistently. Yet to value a positive emphasis does not mean we should assume that everything is positive or that we should never consider negative or ambivalent situations. It is a matter of emphasis, focus, or perspective. It is not easy to maintain a positive outlook in the face of present world conditions or in the face of the personal difficulties we inevitably confront, yet it can help to sustain us.

To accept the value of a positive emphasis does not require a belief that human nature is all good rather than bad; this is too simple. Embracing the positive emphasis for ourselves is closely linked to beginning "in here" and reflecting on our positive resources, celebrating our own positive qualities, and seeing the potential to nourish these positive qualities, using them to cope with negative situations and the possibility of negative qualities in ourselves.

I was initially surprised when some practitioners expressed difficulty in identifying a positive professional experience, but as they described these difficulties, I began to understand. First, some practitioners have few experiences they recall as positive. Second, no experience is completely positive or negative, so the selection must be in general terms. Finally, some practitioners initially feel that celebrating their positive experiences smacks of egotism or narcissism, and is short on humility. In these cases I try to emphasize the distinction between self-absorption and self-awareness. In order to apply "Accentuate the positive" in our own relationships, we need to look for and try to sense the positive in another, often a challenge to our hardened categories of perception. Beyond the basic quality of optimism underlying this value/belief is a willingness to persist in looking for the positive in another which spills over into the general faith in human potential.

Images of this value are primarily transformations from negative to positive — for example, thunderstorm to rainbow, diamond in the rough, silver-lined cloud, and so on. Maintaining optimism is often supported by my sense of humor. I often think of the old joke about the twins, one an optimist and one a pessimist. When the little optimist found a roomful of manure, he exclaimed "There's a pony here somewhere!"

4. Continuity

Continuity and ongoingness reflect the never-ending vitality of the renewal process, the experience of depletion and replenishment, the cyclical nature of renewal. To embrace the value of continuity is to respect the historical continuity of our lives as well as our potential for the future. It is to emphasize the process, the nature of the journey, as well as the product or our arrival at our destination.

The belief in continuity respects the dynamic nature of the human venture, giving meaning to the life force. Using the image of a journey, accepting continuity does not mean that we always travel the shortest distance or arrive in the shortest period of time. The underlying dynamic may seem to involve detours, blind alleys, and getting lost, yet the journey continues (see Chapter Eight). As the image of the rushing stream implies, the cyclical nature of renewal is akin to the cyclical nature of the seasons, to renewal in nature through the rebirth of plants, the generation of new leaves and flowers, and so on. The seasons are both an image and a reality for renewal.

Continuity evokes the quality of patience for me because our lives necessarily proceed through times of difficulty in the journey. Patience is a faith in the life process itself.

5. Contradiction

When I realized that a sense of humor was a means of sensing and experiencing contradiction I also began to sense the importance of this value. As elaborated in the next chapter, I sometimes define research as placing oneself in a position to be surprised. In fact, if you are not in a position to contradict your expectations, you are probably not engaging in research. In research, cumulative understanding comes from accommodating contradictions.

Continuities and discontinuities are both a part of the process of life and renewal. When my wife and I explore a new place by car or on foot, we always expect to get lost; it is a part of the experience. It may be possible to grasp the importance of contradiction by noting that it is how we deal with contradictions that counts. Like every one of the five values in the framework, this one needs qualification; it does not mean that life is completely contradictory, with no pattern, no unity, and no continuity. Rather it means that continuity and contradiction exist side by side, and each needs to be respected.

Overarching human potential

All of the values representing the Spirit of Renewal cohere in the overarching value of human potential, a belief in the vigor, endurance, and resilience of the human spirit. Belief in human potential includes both our own potential to grow and develop and our faith in the capacity of others to do so. It embodies all the qualities described earlier — respect, openness, optimism, patience, and sense of humor —

which come together in the single quality, faith. It means that we respect the possibility for each of us to become more than we are or more than what we may imagine for ourselves. Potential is not limited by age; it applies equally to the elderly and to the young, and perhaps more than anything it requires that we rid ourselves of limited expectations, stereotypes, and fixed predictions. What would this person have to do to surprise me? How can I help that to happen? What would I like to be? What has to happen for that to become reality? These are the kinds of questions that we need to pose when operating from this article of faith.

Burnout and the Spirit of Renewal

Burnout among helping professionals is rapidly reaching crisis proportions. Whether we consider teachers, nurses, daycare workers, social workers, counselors, or others who provide human services, we see evidence that they cannot continue to be responsive to the needs of their clients without some kind of replenishment of their personal energy. For years we treated our natural energy resources as if they were inexhaustible — using and taking, never considering replenishment — but recently we have begun to become aware that our natural resources are not unlimited. Yet, as Seymour Sarason observed in his phrase "the myth of unlimited resources" (1972), we have yet to come to the same understanding of human resources. Just as we faced and continue to face a crisis in natural resources, we now face a crisis in human resources, especially in the helping professions.

In keeping with the theme of burnout, my image of the Spirit of Renewal is that of lighting the spark and keeping the flame alive. For helping professionals whose energy has been depleted, we need to try to help to re-ignite that energy by providing the opportunity and encouragement to re-kindle the spark. For all, we need to consider how to begin treating our human resources in a more respectful way. For this purpose, I propose applying the framework in Table 7 to initiate the Spirit of Renewal within ourselves, within our workplaces, and within our organizations.

In the present situation of dwindling financial resources for the helping professions, many people may find proposals for renewal luxurious. To you I pose the question, How do you propose to deal with the increasing crisis of professional burnout? Initiating the Spirit of Renewal need not be prohibitively expensive; rather, it requires being committed to the belief that by working together we can renew each other and draw on our mutual resources for rejuvenation and replenishment.

As you know, I am not a pessimist. But I must say that from experience with helping professionals, I am convinced that unless there is a dramatic change in attitude and action, the quality of all our services will continue to deteriorate. What

I mean by a change in attitude is illustrated by Seymour Sarason's argument in his newest book, *The Predictable Failure of Educational Reform* (1990a), where he discusses the question, For whom do the schools exist? In contrast to the traditional answer — for students — he argues that the answer must be that the schools are for the students *and* the teachers. In making his case, he points out that a major reason for the failure of earlier attempts at reform was that they did not take into account that teachers, too, were persons, and that they needed opportunities for continuing rejuvenation. The clear implication is that we must arrange our schools in such a way that there will be learning, development, and renewal for all, students and staff alike. This means much more than inserting an occasional Professional Development day; it will mean taking the phrase "Teachers-as-experts" seriously and being committed to providing the time and opportunity which are necessary for sharing as co-creation and for jointly addressing concerns.

I would add to Sarason's critique by noting that the predictable failure inheres in the word "reform" itself, which implies an Outside-in fix to resolve the "problem." We do not need reform; we need renewal as shown in the Spirit of Renewal. In the remainder of this chapter, I will sketch how such a framework might be applied to ourselves, to our work settings, and to our organizations.

Applying the Framework to Ourselves

I invite you to try on the five beliefs for yourself, first bringing out your own images and the qualities that you associate with the five beliefs as discussed earlier. In so doing, you will have a more meaningful basis for experiencing the value of the framework. Of course, you may transform the values, too, or add to them, but first I encourage you to try out the five values in Table 7.

Filling in your own version of Table 7 opens many possibilities. Once you have identified the five qualities you associate with the beliefs, you may reflect on whether these are the central qualities to which you aspire as well as whether there are important omissions. Filling in this framework is the first step in lighting the spark of renewal in yourself, in bringing it into your actions.

How do we bring our beliefs into action? We must tackle this thorny issue if the Spirit of Renewal is to ignite in our lives. Yet we must be cautious to avoid prescriptions. In the following, I summarize the questions I pose to myself to bring these beliefs into my action, to help keep me honest. Some of these questions may work for you, or you may wish to develop other questions. These are not general questions to be answered "yes" or "no"; they are to be raised about all our specific actions throughout the day.

1. Equity of expertise

- Am I conscious of what I know and what I do not know?
- Am I respectful of the knowledge of others?
- Am I willing to listen to an opposite view?

2. Synergy of sharing

- Do I make time and opportunity for sharing?
- Do I listen to others in a way which is helpful to both of us?
- Do I present my views in ways which invite their being transformed and clarified?
- Do I respect another's privacy if they do not wish to share?

3. Positive emphasis

- Do I identify my own positive resources without being overly egotistical, using these resources as a foundation for further growth and development?
- Do I communicate with others by beginning with emphasis on their positive, well-developed qualities?
- Do I use a positive approach in the service of accurate understanding of both myself and others?

4. Continuity

- Do I keep a journal or some other means of recording long-term growth and development, movement along the journey by myself and others?
- Am I patient with myself and others in regard to movement along the journey?
- Am I open to seeing others' perceptions of their own movement?

5. Contradiction

- Do I laugh at myself?
- Can I accept my frailties and imperfections with good humor without losing the possibility of developing further?
- Can I be amused at the impossibility of certain modes of inquiry, for example, psychology, without abandoning my attempt to understand the human venture?

Obviously, I cannot ask myself all of these questions all of the time, yet I find that a judicious sprinkling of them, especially when summarized by a stinger or a tune I can hum, helps me put my beliefs into action. Perhaps some of these questions will work for you; chances are that you will develop others as well. Infusing the Spirit of Renewal into our actions is, of course, an instance of reflection-in-action. Specifically, you will probably need a daily review period to consider your actions in light of your beliefs and to develop some guides for new actions which will be closer to the Spirit of Renewal. I cannot overemphasize the importance of concrete means for representing your qualities/beliefs, for example, a pin depicting your image, a poster which represents the quality which you instill in your actions, a tune which you may hum, such as "Accentuate the Positive," or a stinger. When we are seeking to bring the flame of renewal into our daily actions, we cannot keep an entire framework in our heads to direct our actions; that is why images are so powerful as a guide in this endeavor.

The Spirit of Renewal in Pre-Service Teacher Education

The Spirit of Renewal cannot be "implemented," "delivered," or "put in place"; it can only be ignited from within ourselves and spread to others. In this section, I want to describe how the five basic beliefs might be infused into your work, program, or setting by using the example of pre-service teacher education. The spark of renewal may be lit in many areas — teambuilding, program initiation, mentoring, induction, re-training, and so on — and I hope that this specific discussion will serve as a guide to apply in these other areas.

Renewal may be initiated in a teacher education program by any one or more of those participants in the program — the dean, department head, faculty member, co-operating teacher, or even one or more of the students. The resulting flame will vary in size, depending on who has kindled it: for example, an administrator or a faculty member, as well as by how many have kindled it, but it must begin somewhere.

1. Equity of expertise

In respecting this belief, faculty members would view education students as having a base of experienced knowledge about teaching and learning that is the foundation for their further development as teaching professionals. Specifically, students would bring out their experienced knowledge, in its various forms, as described in Chapter One, as a way to become aware of the implications of their experience and their experienced knowledge for how they are likely to teach. Faculty members would also bring out their experienced knowledge and exemplify in their classes how they put their knowledge into action.

When formal texts are used, faculty would encourage students to raise questions about the author's basis for knowledge, whether it comes from practice, and whether the author gives evidence of putting knowledge into action. Students would also have a chance to use their own experienced knowledge as the base of considering Outside-in theories and possibly extending and developing their own implicit theories.

In their practice teaching, students would be given the opportunity to identify their co-operating teachers' experienced knowledge as well as how it is put into action. In practice teaching, they would be encouraged to reflect on their teaching practice in relation to their experienced knowledge, with an eye to the extent to which their actions are both in accord with their knowledge and validate their implicit theories.

Further, students in practice teaching would have the opportunity to apply the equity of expertise in their practice teaching, that is, to work with their own students in the same ways, respect their knowledge foundation, and build on it to enhance both their own understanding and that of their students in the classroom.

2. Synergy of sharing

Once students have brought out their experienced knowledge, they can share it, as described in the earlier chapters, in pairs or in small groups. The co-creation of sharing would be a major vehicle for further developing their experienced knowledge. Students could also be invited to consider their texts as part of their shared reflection.

Faculty members would participate in the process both by sharing their own experience and experienced knowledge and by giving special attention to the composition of the groups who are sharing. Just as in peer teaching programs, it might be valuable to pair a more experienced student with a less experienced one. As indicated earlier, all of this requires a culture of trust and acceptance, which is greatly facilitated by faculty members' open participation.

The synergy of sharing can be demystified if we compare it to a variation on the model of co-operative learning. Students would be encouraged to use methods of sharing, such as the C-RE-A-T-E Cycle, in their practice teaching so that they might experience the Spirit of Renewal not only in their teacher education classes, but also in their own practice. The more opportunity for renewal, the brighter the flame. My notion of the synergy of sharing in professional education is epitomized by the reflective practicum proposed by Schon (1983; 1987), a powerful means for providing the necessary climate for the synergy of sharing to thrive.

3. Positive emphasis

Being true to a positive emphasis in our actions requires that we directly address the issue of evaluation. I might begin, for example, by discussing with my students both their developed skills and qualities and their underdeveloped ones, indicating the importance of identifying these for ourselves. Next, I would suggest that most of us develop new capacities when we feel supported and not when we feel threatened. Finally, I would suggest that most of us usually know, without being told, when we have a quality or a skill which needs to be developed.

This would set the basis for a positive emphasis as the *initial* focus. Emphasizing the positive will not, of course, in and of itself automatically lead to developing underdeveloped qualities, but it will provide support and confidence to individual students, and encourage them to proceed with their self-development.

The role of evaluation within a Spirit of Renewal framework is the joint responsibility of faculty member and student. The faculty member would invite students to form their own evaluations, with special emphasis on providing evidence for their judgments. Among other things, this procedure would make it clear to students that they do not relinquish their critical faculties by taking a positive approach but rather use their critical awareness in a different climate, one which supports self-evaluation as well as guidance and feedback from faculty members, co-operating teachers, peers, and students.

In their practice teaching, student teachers would apply this value by focusing on their own students' positive or well-developed qualities, and use these as a basis for further development. Faculty members who resist this approach might wish to ask themselves how they developed their knowledge and skills, and whether they did so when they were supported or when they were being criticized for their shortcomings.

4. Continuity

Faculty members and co-operating teachers could exemplify such continuity by describing their own development. Again, this principle flourishes when students also apply it in their practice teaching to their own students.

There is no better means for honoring continuity than by keeping a professional journal. Although their journals will be "for their eyes only," student teachers would be invited to pay special attention to how their initial experienced knowledge became extended, clarified, and validated. Viewed in the context of a journey, professional education calls for marking not only short-term movement but also long-term progress. Part of journal keeping, therefore, might focus on long-term development. It is patience over the long run that sustains us through short-term difficulties. Students would be encouraged to focus their reflections accordingly.

5. Contradiction

Faculty members have an excellent opportunity to exemplify this value by laughing at themselves and their foibles as well as by citing stingers which illustrate the nonlogical, whimsical nature of human affairs (e.g., "The one hallmark of a successful lesson is that it could not be planned in advance"). Of course, faculty members must feel confidence in themselves and their teaching to make fun of themselves, but there is nothing which creates a climate of shared learning more effectively than teachers who reveal their imperfections in a humorous fashion.

Why not a contest for Teaching Bloopers? A climate which acknowledges imperfection and contradiction with a good-natured laugh eases the tensions of performance so that student teachers wind up teaching in a more relaxed, and effective, manner. The key is to laugh at yourself. If students can be encouraged to view their own difficulties as bloopers to be enjoyed and learned from, they will be making the spirit of contradiction, and of humor, their own. And this will serve them well for years to come.

To summarize, the Spirit of Renewal is ignited through our actions. Once it is in our hearts, we extend the spirit to our students through living the Spirit of Renewal; they, in turn, sustain the flame by extending it to their students in their practice teaching. The flame of renewal sheds light and provides warmth to all.

The Renewing Organization

Infusing the Spirit of Renewal in organizations is a challenging, complex topic which could easily provide the scope for an entire book. Two recent books, *The Renewal Factor* (Waterman, 1987) and *Images of Organization* (Morgan, 1986), are especially valuable. These books provide examples from business and industry, many of which come under the category of "excellent" companies. As an example from the education field, where fewer examples are available, I refer to teacher centers which are informal organizations by, for and of the teachers (Hunt, 1989). In discussing each value of the Spirit of Renewal framework with respect to teacher centers, I offer a brief comment on its relevance and potential in renewing educational organizations.

1. Equity of expertise

A renewing organization is horizontal rather than hierarchical to reflect an acknowledgment of the expertise of each individual member. In the renewing organization, persons with greater responsibility are not traditional experts but are responsible for the free flow of resources and expertise among members.

Teacher centers celebrate "teacher as expert." Their ethos is respect for the primacy of practice and the experienced knowledge of practitioners. They provide means for identifying and affirming expertise among the teachers themselves. Most teacher centers are informal, contrasting with the formal hierarchy of school boards and districts which sometimes rival the military in top-down organizational structure.

It is unreasonable to expect the organizational structure of public education to transform itself immediately into the "flat" horizontal structure of the renewing organization, although I note here that this is the approach which excellent companies are adopting. Some hopeful signs are found in schools which promote the equity of expertise and in school-based improvement programs, as discussed at the end of this chapter.

2. Synergy of sharing

The renewing organization provides time and opportunity for members to share and apply their experienced knowledge to organizational concerns. Teamwork is emphasized and rewarded. The climate facilitates the attitudes underlying sharing as co-creation: good will, non-judgmental orientation, respect, openness, and trust. These become a part of the organizational ideology, or value system, which permeates all activities.

In teacher centers, sharing occurs continuously, and they often provide networks for identifying resources among teachers as well as the opportunity for sharing and learning together. Knowledge comes most often from the teachers themselves and is enhanced through the clarification and elaboration in sharing.

Public schools currently endorse co-operative learning as a means to enhance student learning, but this approach, which promotes learning through sharing is not usually carried over to staff renewal. The teacher center ethos occasionally occurs in individual schools, but it has not permeated the structure of public education. Educational administrators might note that when business organizations initiate opportunities for sharing, the results are not only increased job satisfaction, but also enhanced product quality.

3. Positive orientation

The renewing organization celebrates the well-developed qualities of each member. Groups may be organized with members whose expertise complements one another. They build on success, and sustain their optimism and good will through mutual support and co-operation.

One of the most important contributions of teacher centers is that they provide a means of restoring confidence and empowering individual teachers through celebrating their small victories and their positive professional experiences. They may help teachers cope with excessive demands and come to terms with the fact they cannot do everything for every student.

Again, public education presents a dilemma. While students are viewed ideally, as full of potential, teachers are usually seen in terms of their deficits and weaknesses and as needing remediation which in turn produces demoralization. Public education must begin by treating teachers with the same positive orientation that is extended to students.

4. Continuity

The renewing organization emerges from its own history, from its integrity, which derives from living by its values. It respects long-range goals as well as short-term targets. Persons in a renewing organization may keep journals of their work so they can gain from their own and others' stories, taking note of whether adherence to organizational beliefs is associated with movement toward organizational goals.

Teacher centers provide an opportunity for teachers to stop and consider the longer-term goals of development, their own and those of their students. They provide a haven temporarily removed from the demands of the world of action where reflection is impossible. One might say, tongue in cheek, that public education has too much continuity if we think of continuity as consistency, since public schools are very slow to change. However, this is a limited vision of continuity which must be combined with contradiction so that we reflect on what has worked and what has failed in the past.

5. Contradiction

In attending to individual and organizational development and growth, the renewing organization must also alert to discontinuities and contradiction, to what Gareth Morgan (1989) called "faultlines" which may indicate areas which need more attention.

Teachers confront hundreds of contradictions in their classrooms every day. Teacher centers provide an opportunity for teachers to consider these contradictions — for example, of gender, ethnicity, and ability or disability — to jointly consider what might be done, or perhaps what cannot be dealt with at the moment.

The Renewing Organization as an Organizational Culture

Another way to view renewing organizations is in terms of the seven dimensions describing organizational cultures as proposed by Schein (1990).

1. Relation to environment

A renewing organization is open to its environment, seeks harmony, but is capable of coping with contradictions. In the case of school boards and schools, they provide networks for feedback and interaction with their various employees, clients, and stakeholders.

2. The nature of human activity

The renewing organization strongly emphasizes resources and responsibilities based on a fundamental belief in the potential of members of the organization. Norms of respect and openness are practiced and rewarded. Activity is organized in order to tap the resources and knowledge of members within the organization as far as possible rather than relying on outside experts.

3. The nature of reality and truth

In a renewing organization, truth is approached through sharing the experienced knowledge of group members which is then put into action for verification. A renewing organization seeks truth through a specific combination of wisdom (in the form of individual member's experienced knowledge) and social consensus (through sharing) which is put to test in practice. It is vital that time and opportunity be provided for bringing out, sharing and applying experienced knowledge.

4. The nature of time

The renewing organization addresses the nature of time with the quality of patience and an emphasis on the continuous, long-term process of growth and development. The organization sees itself in relation to the past as a foundation for continuing development. The emphasis is on the continuing process of renewal which includes energy depletion and replenishment over both the short and long run. Members of the organization are encouraged to maintain records or journals to make their continuous development.

5. The nature of human nature

A renewing organization views human nature as imperfect but perfectible. It respects the enormous untapped resources of its members; it holds optimism about the possibility of developing our resources beyond our own or the organization's expectation. This belief in human potential, given organizational support, is the keystone to the culture of a renewing organization.

6. The nature of human relationships

The renewing organization is based on collegial participation. Having committed itself to the equity of expertise and the synergy of sharing, it provides time and opportunity for group members to bring out their untapped resources and put them into action. In a school setting, such beliefs and practices need to be initiated in classrooms as well as at the administrative level.

7. Homogeneity vs. diversity

For a renewing organization, diversity provides the contradictions which spark the energy of renewal. Accommodating diversity is perhaps one of the most difficult challenges in the world today. The renewing organization honors diversity and provides opportunities for capturing its energy.

Characterizing a renewing organization along these dimensions provides a tentative sketch of what such an organization might be like, but provides no hint of how to create a renewing organization. Unless we are dealing with the creation of a new organization, the challenge is how to modify the organizational culture of an organization in the direction of renewal.

I found a recent recommendation by Gareth Morgan (1989) helpful. Reflecting his fondness for images and metaphors, Morgan recommends that human resource developers operate like "termites" within their organizations. By this he does not mean only "boring from within," but rather emulating termite activity which consists of building tunnels and creating structures which are unrelated to a master plan. Morgan recommends that the facilitator "start small," without a master plan for reorganization, keeping an eye out for areas within the organization which are acting on the desired beliefs. Then the facilitator should try to encourage these areas and their activities from within. To facilitate renewal within an organization, therefore, we need to be alert to individuals who exemplify the Spirit of Renewal and to encourage them.

The Spirit of Renewal in School-Based Improvement

As I completed the final draft of this book, I undertook to work with the staff of a Toronto high school. The principal had invited me to discuss the possibility of collaboration after he had read an early draft of this book. He had been especially taken by the idea of the untapped resources among staff members.

At our first meeting, I learned that this inner city high school served a variety of ethnic students as well as a large number of special needs students (200 of the 750 students were so designated). The staff members included counselors, translators, and support staff as well as classroom teachers. Further, I learned that four areas of concern had been identified by the staff: (1) student evaluation, (2) peer mentoring, (3) student learning style, and (4) co-operative learning. We discussed possibilities for a school-based initiative which would allow the staff to learn more about these four areas.

At our next meeting, we were joined by two department heads and two consultants from the board office, and we began to develop a tentative plan which covered the next 12 months. Prior to a two-day workshop in January, all staff members were asked to select one of the four topics to work on. Based on their choices, they were assigned to four "topic teams" which formed the organizational basis for the initiative; topic teams met monthly after the workshops to plan professional development presentations for the following fall. Thus, the professional development activities for the fall were the responsibility of staff members who had committed themselves to share their resources with the rest of their colleagues. Each topic team was lead by a consultant from the board office who had some experience with the topic. The District Superintendent was very supportive of the initiative and provided the possibility of a second day for the January workshop (he attended the first day himself).

On the first day, in the morning, staff members who were seated in topic teams brought out their experienced knowledge by using methods described earlier in this book. In the afternoon, they tried the C-RE-A-T-E Cycle.

On the second day, staff met in four separate rooms by topic teams led by the board consultant. Each team brought out their own resources and knowledge about their specific topic — for example, student evaluation. The consultant provided "outside" information on the topic at this meeting. Each staff member was encouraged to begin an individual initiative on the topic — for example, work out a specific means of evaluating one student — which they developed through the C-RE-A-T-E Cycle format.

Following the two-day workshop, monthly meetings were held. These began with an informal luncheon for all followed by two-hour meeting by topic teams in which plans were developed for how staff wished to present their ideas in the forthcoming professional development meetings in the fall.

Let's consider this initiative in terms of the five values in the Spirit of Renewal framework. First, the initiative began with the principal's belief in the equity of expertise (the untapped resources of his staff), and it was facilitated by workshops in which staff brought out their inner wisdom which they used as the foundation exploring their areas of concern. Second, the value of sharing was acknowledged throughout the initiative at every phase — from the C-RE-A-T-E Cycle to the topic teams, (which usually worked in small groups), to the final presentations. Third, positive emphasis was maintained throughout, explicitly through focusing on positive professional experiences and implicitly through the luncheon get-togethers which celebrated the staff and their students. Fourth, continuity was the basic foundation for the topic team meetings and for their presentations. Continuity was also important in each staff member's attempt to apply the topic individually. Fifth, no initiative is perfect, so what were the contradictions? A few staff members did not feel that they had been consulted in the plans, a concern which contradicts respect for the equity of expertise. This was dealt with on the second day of the workshop. A few other staff members indicated that they were not interested in working on the topic team: a concern which contradicts the motions of synergy and the continuity of interests, so the activity of exploring these topics had to be identified as voluntary. Once these issues of choice and of voluntary participation had been addressed, the initiative seemed to move along very well.

CHAPTER SEVEN

Research as Renewal

The growing interest in qualitative inquiry in education represents more than a mere refining of existing models of inquiry. It represents the beginning of a new way of thinking about the nature of knowledge and how it can be created.

Elliott Eisner

When those of you who are not researchers read the word "research" in this chapter, you may feel that this is a very specialized topic which is likely to be uninteresting and/or incomprehensible. Yet, research plays a vital role in our lives through public opinion surveys, evaluation studies of various kinds of social services and through "basic research" and inquiry into human affairs. My major theme in this chapter is to remind you that inquiry into human affairs is itself part of human affairs. As George Kelly (1955) put it, psychology is a unique discipline because the researcher/theorist is both a perpetrator of theories about the human condition and a participant in it.

To acknowledge that inquiry into human affairs is itself a part of human affairs is also to acknowledge that the results of inquiry are influenced by the intentions and expectations of both the researcher and the persons being researched, as well as by the relationship between them. Researchers in human affairs are often reluctant to admit the human side of their activity since it erodes their detached role as "social scientists" which is the basis of their research expertise, a belief borrowed from the physical scientists. Calling their work science cannot erase the fact that researchers are persons, too, and researchers' failure to acknowledge this is a major reason for the irrelevance and lack of practical value of their research.

Why should non-researchers be concerned with what sounds like a technical issue in human affairs research, usually referred to as social science? Not only does social science evaluation research cost taxpayers money, but the results often support major policy decisions in social service and educational planning. So bring back your Critic and consider such research from the standpoint that researchers are persons, too.

Take as a specific example the research evaluating daycare as opposed to childcare in the home by a parent (or parents). Put your Critic to work on these questions:

- What are the underlying beliefs of those conducting research?
- Do they favor or oppose daycare?
- Do they have children in daycare?
- Who is sponsoring the research and what is their stake in the results?
- What would be the response of the sponsors or the researchers to findings which are opposite to their beliefs and expectations, for example that daycare is inferior to care at home?

Let's push this example a little further.

- How does the researcher see daycare workers in terms of renewal and burnout?
- Why are these workers willing to provide continuous and responsive care for children who are not part of their own families?
- What conditions might be necessary for daycare workers to avoid burnout?
- How can we avoid the error of the "myth of unlimited resources" in daycare?

Perhaps the most important question to pose to our Critic is:

- To what extent is the researcher going through the motions to create the illusion of objectivity, while the true aim is to verify social/educational policy which has already been determined?

I do not mean that researchers are dishonest, but that they simply may not be open to the surprise of contradictory findings.

Proposing an Inside-out approach to research is not novel. My ideas are in the spirit of developments of the past 20 years which have legitimized bringing the researcher into the research process as a participant in the human venture. Such research approaches may be called non-traditional, phenomenological, ethnographic, qualitative or collaborative research. I will call these approaches "Research-as-renewal" because I use the Spirit of Renewal framework in Table 7 to derive their characteristics as shown in Table 9.

Table 9

Imbuing a Spirit of Renewal into Research

Value/Belief	Research as renewal	Related Quality
Equity of Expertise	Both researcher and researched are participants in the human venture	Respect
Synergy of Sharing	Research as the negotiation of intentions of researcher and researched	Openness
Positive Emphasis	Research as portraying what we may be	Optimism
Continuity	Research as increased personal understanding	Patience
Contradiction	Research as openness to surprise	Sense of humor/surprise

Below I discuss the five images of Research-as-renewal to illustrate the nature of this kind of inquiry. It is unlikely that any single research project will embrace all five perspectives. Nevertheless, I hope they provide some understanding of why research sometimes fails as well as some new perspectives for planning future research.

Researcher and Researched as Persons in the Human Venture

Equity of expertise in research means that researchers view themselves and those researched as co-participants in the human venture, each having experienced knowledge which is to be respected as contributing to the inquiry. To discuss how the researcher's assumptions about human nature influence research, I extend MacMurray's (1961) idea that persons may be viewed as *"persons,"* as *"organisms,"* or as *"objects"* (see Table 10).

As Table 10 shows, we are not only persons, but also organisms and objects. As objects, we are subject to the laws of physical motion so that if we fall, for example, the velocity of our fall follows the laws of physics governing falling objects. As organisms, we are subject to the principles which govern lower organisms such as our need for food and water. Finally, we are persons; we are participants in the human venture and our actions are intentional, and we may be aware of and report these intentions.

How researchers choose to view those researched profoundly influences their research findings. When researchers treat persons as objects, they learn *only* about their physical movement as physical objects. When researchers treat persons as organisms, they learn *only* about their basic needs and their reflexes. However, when researchers treat those whom they research as persons, then they are more likely to uncover understandings which are relevant to the human condition,and therefore contain practical value.

Check this assumption by considering you own experience. Have you ever participated in an experiment in which you were treated as an organism — that is, as a subject? If so, chances are you felt powerless and tried to figure out what it was that the experimenter wanted so that you could give the desired response and get out of the situation as quickly as possible. Consider how the results of research are colored by ignoring the subject's personhood, intentions, and perceptions. More specifically, always ask the questions, Why were those researched participating in the research? What do they get out of it? Does it have any perceived benefit for them? Do they have any reason to be forthcoming and honest with the researcher?[6]

---

6. The introduction of ethical reviews and informed consent has limited the tendency to dehumanize research subjects but a great deal of research continues in this tradition.

Table 10
How assumptions about human nature influence research

When those researched are viewed as	The researcher is called	Those researched are called	Relation between researcher and researched	Focus of research
Persons	Researcher	Participants	Persons-in-relation; reciprocal	Intentional action
Organisms	Experimenter (E)	Subjects (Ss)	E runs Ss	Behavior
Objects	Experimenter (E)	Objects	E observes objects	Physical movement

The three images of human nature depicted in Table 10 have related implications for the role of the researcher. When researchers are experimenters, they are detached from the human venture and maintain an impersonal objectivity. Yet their research, by its nature, prevents understanding of the human situation.

If applied research is to be authentic and relevant, researchers must first accept their own personhood, their co-participation in the human venture they seek to understand. As mentioned earlier, the failure to acknowledge this is probably the largest single reason for the failure of social science research to influence practice. When applied research emulates the physical sciences, the personal intentions of researchers, which are the driving force behind inquiry, are assumed to be negative forces which need to be controlled or eliminated. Certainly researchers must consider their intentions as they conduct their research, but not by deluding themselves about the elimination of their intentions. Our personal intentions, along with the related perceptions and actions which flow from them, are our most powerful and sensitive means for recording and interpreting our research. As researchers we need to be aware of our personal intentions, perceptions, and actions, but to try to eliminate them as "experimenter bias" is to cut us off from our perceptual antennae and our capacity to make meaning, both precious qualities of ourselves. The idea of "eliminating personal bias" is a misguided illusion whose effect is to guarantee the irrelevance of the research. If an investigation requires the elimination of "bias," let a computer record the results.

A good rule for researchers is "Become the first participant in your study." Whether this means completing a questionnaire, being observed in your practice, or being interviewed, beginning with yourself is almost certain to increase your sensitivity to the participants in your research. For example, Sharon Bray (1986) has explored the value of video feedback for faculty members to improve their teaching. She began her study by videotaping herself as she described the research participants; then she played the video and invited feedback on her own teaching. As Table 9 indicates, the best way for researchers to communicate their belief in the equity of expertise is through respect, specifically by conveying the attitude that they will learn a great deal from the participants in this research and that what they will learn will be accessible to participants.

Research as the Negotiation of Intentions

Researchers usually enter the research initiative with a clear idea of what they want from the transaction, yet such is not usually the case for participants, who have intentions, too. Therefore, researchers need to talk with participants prior to the final development of their design in order to discover how the research can be meaningful for them. In such preliminary discussion, the researcher poses to the prospective participant the question, Having described my proposed research and what I hope to learn, how might the research be presented to you so that you would find it potentially valuable and would wish to participate? In short, the researcher becomes the learner, seeking feedback from potential participants.

Giving prior consideration to the intentions of those researched is much more than a device to "motivate" participants; it acknowledges the need to consider the intentions of both parties and to negotiate a mutually satisfactory arrangement. Often participants' primary concern is that they will receive specific and individual feedback following their participation. Sometimes, in addition to providing feedback, researchers may provide extrinsic rewards. Brathwaite (1988), for example, provided training in microcomputers in addition to feedback about the research to the teachers who participated in her study. However, extrinsic rewards are usually secondary to the intrinsic satisfaction participants gain from the activity. Imagine that you were being asked to participate in a research project. Realizing your time is valuable, what questions would you ask? What would be necessary for you to agree to participate? How important would extrinsic rewards be in your decision?

In formal research such as a doctoral thesis, the negotiation of intentions is spelled out in a consent form which participants sign, yet the spirit of mutually shared intentions transcends a formal agreement because it continues throughout the research process and forms the basis of the research relationship. Put another way, the Spirit of Renewal cannot be completely expressed in a formal agreement such as a consent form.

It is probably too optimistic to assume that the researcher and participant will be able to work together in a spirit of sharing as co-creation described in Chapter Four, yet this should be the goal. The more their relationship approaches sharing as co-creation, the more meaningful and valuable will be the results of the inquiry.

Research as Portraying What We May Be

The hallmark of *applied* research in human affairs is its practical value: improvement of the human condition, whether improvement takes the form of facilitating growth and development or improving human services to accomplish these goals. To achieve these practical aims, applied research inquiry needs to explore the potential of development and how to facilitate bringing potential to reality. Yet such is rarely the case. Too often applied social science research simply reinforces and verifies the status quo, of what we have been rather than our potential, or in Ferrucci's indelible book title *What We May Be* (1982).

This preoccupation with past capacity rather than future potential is illustrated by the nature and use of intelligence testing in North America. IQ testing initially gained legitimacy here because the IQ was not supposed to change. Psychometrically the IQ is reliable and consistent. Humanistically it is a personal prison. Not only does IQ testing fail to deal with potential, but it also regards future development which changes the person's score relative to others as a defect of the test, a sign of unreliability

Contrast the traditional view of intelligence with the work of Schafer-Simmern described by Sarason (1990b). Schafer-Simmern worked with mentally handicapped persons to find out about their capacity for artistic expression through painting and drawing. It is important to note that he approached his work with the belief that every person, no matter how disabled, has the potential for artistic expression. His patience was rewarded. These developmentally disabled persons, whom traditional wisdom would say were incapable of anything like artistic expression, were quite creative and artistic when given the opportunity and allowed to work in an environment in which their potential was an article of faith.

A similar example is found in the work of John Sumarah (1985) who also worked with developmentally disabled persons. Among other things, he was interested in exploring their potential for imagery, and he found, as did Schafer-Simmern, that when one believed in their potential, treated them accordingly with gentleness and patience, they were quite capable of rich imagery. Pause for a moment to consider the implications of these results with developmentally disabled people: Why have we failed to acknowledge this potential? How can we deal with the fixed stereotypes underlying traditional views of their limited potential? What might happen if they were encouraged?

I selected examples from work with severely disabled people to emphasize the untapped potential in everyone. Research as what we may be opens many avenues for dealing with what we think of as limited human resources. But let me note two ironies before citing further specific examples. First, it is Soviet psychologists, for example, Vygotsky, who have led the way in exploring the extension of human potential, a curious state of affairs in terms of the ethos of the Soviet Union and the espoused ethos in Canada and the United States. Second, traditional researchers have acknowledged the influence of the belief in human potential through what Rosenthal and Jacobson called *Pygmalian in the Classroom* (1968) which refers to the influence of the teacher's or experimenter's expectations on the performance of the student in the classroom or on the subject in an experiment. Curiously, however, rather than taking these results as evidence for the importance of investigating human potential, they were regarded as "error variance" to be avoided and controlled. It is quite appropriate to control "experimenter bias" in research or the effects of certain drugs, for example, through placebos and "double blind" designs, but not so in research in human affairs, where researchers' positive expectations are essential to discovering human potential.

How human potential is fostered by "accentuating the positive" is illustrated by Ardra Cole's (1987) thesis. She explored the process of teachers' spontaneous adaptation to their students, and specifically, the split-second intuitive matching which epitomizes excellent teaching. In her intensive work with two teachers, Cole used their previously evoked personal images to record their images-in-action from classroom observations. She summarized her impressions in weekly reports which were presented to the teacher. Her summaries focused on the teacher's successful adaptations and use of their images-in-action. Her intent was to record specific documentation from the teacher's own perspective which would both provide support and stimulate reflection. In short, she accentuated the positive.

Note that the emphasis in Cole's research contrasts with many supervisory approaches which, though partially positive, usually conclude with negative criticism, pointing to deficiencies. What was the effect of unconditional positive acceptance on the teachers in Cole's study? At the conclusion of the research, both teachers (1) expressed appreciation for the wholehearted acceptance and support, (2) indicated their awareness of areas in their teaching which needed to be developed, and (3) noted that the support gave them confidence to begin working on areas which needed further development. These teachers, like most of us, were aware of their underdeveloped qualities and skills, and did not need further reminders which would serve to discourage them. What they needed was support — a belief in what they might be — which would enable them to work toward achieving their potential. In your own experience, have you developed toward your potential when you were reminded of your faults, or when you were encouraged to move toward your potential on your own terms?

In all of these examples (Schafer-Simmern, Sumarah, and Cole), there is an underlying and ever-present belief in "what we may be." In advocating that researchers accentuate the positive to gain an understanding of human potential, I do not imply that everything is possible and that every person can and will develop every quality. The self-fulfilling prophecy applies to those who believe in human potential as well as to those who do not, but it works in different ways. The restricted prophesy of traditional researchers who believe that "the best predictor of future behavior is past behavior" is likely to be fulfilled, but they will *never* learn anything of the possibilities of human potential. By contrast, researchers whose work is guided by the principle of what we might be, open themselves to the possibility of learning about human potential. Ironically, when their prophecies are fulfilled, they unveil a past of human potential. In short, they *may* learn about human potential and development, while traditional researchers *can never* learn about it.

Research as Increased Personal Understanding

As are all forms of renewal, research is an ongoing, continuous process. Research-as-renewal means an expansion of researchers' experienced knowledge through inquiry. Researchers begin their inquiry by bringing out their own experienced knowledge about their topics, that is, the phenomena they are studying. The inquiry therefore provides an opportunity for researchers to enhance and extend their experienced knowledge and understanding.

In many of the examples I cite below, researchers began their research with themselves by describing their personal experience and/or citing their own experienced knowledge. Using this as a foundation, researchers may record their research journey through keeping journals. Such journals are valuable in providing researchers with an indication of movement and development. Keeping a journal of one's research journey also facilitates your openness to surprise (the next principle) by documenting your tentative expectations.

Viewing research as the expansion of the researcher's experienced knowledge offers a much different view from the traditional physical science version of research accepted by traditional social science. In contrast to this version of research which calls for controlling or eliminating the researcher's beliefs, Research-as-renewal calls for making the researcher's beliefs explicit and bringing them to the center of the inquiry. For example, Brathwaite (1988) made her assumptions about teaching and learning explicit at the outset of her research, and she looked for confirmation or disconfirmation in her interviews and observations. Most of her assumptions were confirmed, though some were altered and expanded upon through her inquiry. When researchers make their beliefs explicit, they are also responsible for indicating how they are "putting their beliefs to the test," that is, how are they opening themselves to disconfirmation and how will they accommodate it. This takes us to the final principle.

Research as Openness to Surprise

I once wrote, half in jest, "In theories of human affairs, psychological theorists can elevate their beliefs to the level of scientific truth" (Hunt, 1983, p. 12). As discussed earlier, researchers' intentions, values, and expectations are always an important influence in their research. Their beliefs affect every phase of their research — its design, selection of participants, and especially interpretation of results. The challenge in researchers' opening themselves to surprise, therefore, is to transcend this human tendency to validate our own beliefs. I suggest several specific ways to meet this challenge in the next section, and here will only touch on some possibilities.

One of the most effective ways to open yourself to surprise is to include in your research some participants who are either very different from the other participants or who hold beliefs which are clearly different from your own. This is not always easy to accomplish and requires respect and openness in negotiating participation. For example, Bradley Bernstein (1978) intensively studied four teachers who were trying out dramatic exercises in their special education classes. He took pains to include one teacher who had initially been resistant to introducing these approaches in her classroom and whose basic beliefs were at odds with his own. The results were a much more credible rendition of these innovative classroom practices. But it is not only in selecting participants that researchers manifest their openness to surprise; it is manifested in the methodology as well. Does the interview and/or observation schedule allow for, indeed even encourage, unexpected results?

The New Three R's in Research: Specific Suggestions

The remainder of this chapter is devoted to researchers who are initiating and carrying out Research-as-renewal. Although I have written it primarily for doctoral students who are conducting their thesis research, I hope that it will also be helpful to researchers in general and "consumers" of research who wish to become better informed.

Table 11
Research-as-renewal vs. Traditional research

Research-as-renewal (Inside-out)	Traditional research (Outside-in)
Researchers begin with themselves (Reflexive)	Researchers begin with logical theories and literature review (Objective)
Researchers listen to and consider intentions of potential participants (Responsive)	Researchers treat all subjects in same impersonal manner (Fixed)
Researcher and participants form collaborative relation (Reciprocal)	One-way relationship; E runs Ss (Unilateral)

The New Three R's, as introduced in Table 3 (p. 31), suggest another way to portray Research-as-renewal: Reflexivity, Responsiveness, and Reciprocality. Table 11 summarizes their implications for researchers, and contrasts this Inside-out approach with traditional Outside-in research, (see "How to Be Your Own Best Researcher," in Hunt, 1987, pp. 117-120). The New Three R's involve researchers in a three-step sequence whereby they (1) begin with themselves by bringing out their previous experience in research and with their research topic, (2) interview potential participants to learn more about their intentions and perceptions, and (3) on the basis of interviews, negotiate a mutually acceptable research relationship.

In the following sections I elaborate this sequence and add other specific suggestions which I make to doctoral students in my research seminar. Examples cited are from those doctoral students in the Focus on Teaching Program who are experienced practitioners conducting research for their dissertations.

1. Bringing out your attitudes to research

The foundation for Research-as-renewal is researchers' awareness of their underlying beliefs, attitudes, and perceptions regarding research in general and their topic in particular. The first step in developing such reflexive awareness (the First R) is to bring out your experienced knowledge about research by recalling your experience not so much as a researcher, but as someone being researched, whether as a voluntary participant or an unwilling subject. The exercise described below is aimed at bringing out this kind of experienced knowledge.

The exercise involves using the Kolb Cycle as an interview guide. Working in pairs, your partner first asks you to recall an experience in which you were researched, and in this case the experience does not need to have been positive. Your partner then, acting as interviewer and recording your responses on tape, invites you to go through the four steps of the Kolb Cycle described in the exercise in Chapter One. After spending a few moments recalling your experience in the research situation as completely as possible, you then jot down the highlights. Using these highlights, you develop some ideas about what the experience meant to you and why this was so. Finally, you review the experience in order to derive some guidelines or principles for conducting your own research in a way that is true to your own beliefs and values.

This cycle can be repeated for other specific experiences related to participation in experiments and/or surveys or in field-testing new programs. The purpose in all cases is to bring out the person's underlying beliefs. One doctoral researcher had previously been treated like an inanimate object in a study, which of course created considerable frustration and negative feelings. Hoping not to repeat this in conducting her own research, she was concerned to develop a proposal which would treat those being researched as persons with intentions and feelings.

As indicated, the Kolb Cycle interview enables researchers to derive specific guidelines/criteria for developing their research proposals. In another example, the doctoral researcher developed such criteria as (1) the researcher should take account of the needs of those being researched, (2) he or she should attempt to build a trusting relationship with those being researched, and (3) he or she should give feedback as soon as possible. These principles are similar to those advocated earlier in this chapter, but they have more meaning when researchers bring them out for themselves and base them on their own experience.

As noted in Table 11, the traditional role of the researcher is to "run the subjects," which conjures up an image of a mechanical function such as an assembly line. What are alternative images of the researcher's role? Mary Beattie (1991) described her intensive collaboration with an experienced teacher in musical terms — "making music" and "playing together" — rich images which opened new perspectives on their collaboration: "What shall we play today?" "I seem to be a little out of tune," and so on.

2. Defining and refining your research topic

What will be the topic of your doctoral thesis? This seemingly simple question stymies doctoral students because they often have had little experience in posing research questions and hold enormously unrealistic ideas about the scope of their topic (initially they want to "cover the world"). In my thesis seminar, I suggest people develop their intention statement as follows: (1) use the form of personal intention ("I want to . . .") rather than the more traditional third person passive form for stating their research objective ("The purpose of the research is . . ."), (2) jot down their topic in the form of an intention statement in no more than 25 words on a 3 x 5 card, (3) for those who do not have any idea about their topic, to reverse Yogi Berra's well-known stinger, "It ain't over 'til it's over," to "You won't get started until you begin," and, finally, (4) get a pack of 3 x 5 cards so that they can continually revise their intention statement as they reflect, share it with others, read reports, and talk to potential participants. The aim here is to increase precision and clarity as they revise the intention statement.

I describe their thesis process as their thesis journey (see next chapter on the inner journey) in which the intention statement is their gyroscope guiding their movement. The intention statement guides by pointing the way through design, method, and interpretation as well as by indicating what is not being studied.

Another aim of the intention statement exercise is to raise awareness of the form of intention statements or research objectives. I suggest to students that when they read a research report or a doctoral thesis, they try to find the statement which summarizes the purpose of the research and record it so that they will accumulate a number of such statements. Once they have collected several intention statements/

objectives, the idea is to look closely at their form:

- What verb is used — for example, "to investigate," "to explore," "to evaluate," "to characterize," etc.?
- What are the related methodological implications of these different verbs?
- Is this object of inquiry (i.e., the phenomenon) described in abstract conceptual terms or specific practical terms? For example, "self-efficacy" and "attribution" as contrasted with "feelings of success" and "personal understanding"?
- Are proposed participants included in the statement of purpose?
- Does the statement include reference to methodology — for example, "a qualitative approach to," "by factor analysis" (My own personal recommendation is that the purpose not include reference to methodology.)

Reading several such statements and becoming aware of their form and lexicon helps doctoral students frame their own statements more precisely as well as become aware of the differential implications of research which is intended to "explore" as opposed to "evaluate." I sometimes use the image of exploring and mapping territory to clarify the most appropriate verb for a specific topic. If the topic has only rarely been studied (unexplored territory and unmapped terrain), then the verb "explore," with its related implication of providing a general "lay of the land," may be appropriate. However, if the topic has been extensively studied (detailed maps are available), then the verb, the methodology, and level of understanding must be geared accordingly — for example "to identify specific. . . ."

The aim of continual revision and refining of intention statements is to evolve one which will guide the research through every phase — rationale, relation to literature, methodology, collection of material, analysis, and implications. In addition to this gyroscopic function, the intention statement should also be comprehensible to others, especially potential participants. Although this sounds simple, the evolution of an intention statement often requires several months. For example, one doctoral researcher began with the statement, "I want to look at how teachers experience the creative thinking process." Several dozen cards later he had transformed it to "I want to observe the effect which bringing out their implicit theories of creativity has on the work of teachers and managers."

3. Bringing out your implicit theories about your topic

Most of the doctoral students in our program are experienced practitioners, many of whom select a research topic from their work setting. In the early meetings of our research seminar, I often pose the question, "Can we conduct research on a topic/ phenomenon which we have not directly experienced?" When researchers begin with themselves and their experienced knowledge and view the inquiry as increasing their understanding of the topic (see Table 9), the answer to the question is likely to be no. But this is not the whole story. Often when we discuss this issue, someone will ask such provocative questions as, "How can we understand and conduct inquiry into another place (culture) or another time (history) we have not directly experienced?" But we are not concerned with history, geography, or distant cultures; we are concerned with human affairs in our own time and place, and here the issue is more challenging.

In any case, doctoral students do occasionally choose to study phenomena which they themselves have not directly experienced, and here they must rely on related experiences or vicarious experience in reading about the phenomenon.

The exercise for bringing out your implicit theories about your research topics is once again using the Kolb Cycle as an interview guide which begins with a specific experience related to the topic. A researcher who has no direct experience with the topic must begin with a related experience. The exercise proceeds in the same fashion through the four steps described above to bring out your attitudes to research. However, here you select a positive experience involving the phenomenon/topic you want to study, and the emphasis is on *why* you think this positive experience occurred or your understanding of what happened. The exercise provides you with the seed of your implicit theories about your practice, so it represents the beginning sketches of your underlying beliefs about your research topic.

Brader Brathwaite (1988) called this process "unveiling the researcher's perceptions" and she described its benefits as follows:

> I was convinced that reflecting on my past experiences in different social and educational milieux, especially in Trinidad, would provide grounding and orientation for my immediate assignment, as well as produce a personal frame of reference from which I can receive input from the prospective participants in the study. Somehow, my past would have to blend with my present in order to provide the coherence which I sought. In preparation for this, I had written an extensive text, almost an autobiography of my learning experiences. I eventually called that text my "chalice" of experiences. (p. 26)

4. Bringing out your image of your research

Using the same positive experience with your research topic that served to identify your implicit theories, you can proceed to evoke your personal image(s) of the topic. Images of the research topic are sometimes quite distinct from one's image of being a researcher, and in other cases they coalesce into the same image. In the following example, the researcher evolved three different images:

1)   The Dolphin represents my practice: a balanced wave-like movement between the conscious and the unconscious, the "ordinary" consensual state of consciousness, and the "non-ordinary" altered state of con-

sciousness, the outer and the inner world. These two worlds are represented by air and water.

2)   The Weaver of Opposites represents my way of learning and sharing knowledge by linking seemingly disparate and conflicting elements into a dynamic whole.

3)   The Vortex represents my process of inquiry. It suggests a descent into the depths, "hitting the bottom," a release, an ascent, and expansion along widening spirals.

In other cases, the researcher may transform and modify the original images:

After working with my image of empty pages, I have been able to attribute more meaning to it. I now see the empty book as a challenge and an opportunity to fill it in the manner I choose. I can now see that there may be as many theories for my phenomena as there are pages in a book, and that each page (i.e., theory) can contribute to the whole by adding or taking away from the previous pages (i.e., theories). It has been a relief to believe that my approach can be as significant as any other. It has taken the pressure off in many ways.

Sometimes, the image works to the cycle of research:

I am walking through a field scattering seeds on fertile soil which has been turned over carefully and cleaned of weeds and debris. The work is painstaking but it is also pleasant because it involves savoring the smells, sights, and sounds of the countryside. The sun is nurturing me and I can feel that it is doing the same for the seeds as they nestle into the earth. Soon the rain will fall, moistening the seeds and encouraging them to sprout. The rain and the sun provide the right conditions for the sprouts to burst out of their casing and reach skyward. Then as the seeds become tall blades of grain the cycle will be repeated at some other time perhaps by some other person.

Since I project my own image of the development and completion of a doctoral thesis as a journey, it is not surprising that many researchers evoke similar images:

The use of images has sustained me throughout the term. In the Fall term, I equated my thesis journey with a trolley car in San Francisco, with no special destination. The change of images since then has encouraged me to realize that I am making progress in spite of many doubts. Using images in conjunction with the more practical aspects of thesis writing provides an interesting balance of the fanciful with the practical.

The next example illustrates how the rejection of an image can be liberating. I often use an imagery exercise which invites participants to evoke their "image of wisdom." Sometimes, the initial image is stereotyped and false, as this researcher discovered:

> Implicit in my resistance to the image of the sage was resistance to the notion of a psychologist as an all-knowing director of people's lives, and as a completely objective researcher. The traditional appearance of a sage with flowing robes seems very compatible with "mainstream" psychology. My resistance to the image is therefore in concert with my resistance to particular aspects of mainstream psychology. Moreover, the ensuing clarity that was evident in my view from the mountaintop was in concert with my acceptance of the notion that my research would proceed from my own point of view. Thus, unlike the sage, I do not know everything, nor can I be completely objective. Rather, I increasingly understand my own point of view and the ways in which it is similar or dissimilar to others' perspectives and I know that it is okay to approach my work in this way.

One colleague found the image of Francis Bacon to be valuable:

> "Those who have handled sciences have been either men of experiment or men of dogma. The men of experiment are like the ant; they collect and they use; the reasoners resemble the spiders who make cobwebs out of their own substance. But the bee takes the middle course; it gathers its material from the folowers of the garden and of the fields but transforms and digests it by a power of its own."

Once doctoral students have brought out their implicit theories and images about their research and their topics, they can pool their resources using the C-RE-A-T-E Cycle (Chapter Five) which leads to a more focused version of the thesis support group.

5. Getting in touch with the phenomenon

Doctoral researchers often believe that they must develop their thesis proposals without leaving their desk or the library. In the traditional view, once a proposal has been logically derived and appropriately positioned within the literature, the proposal is approved and the researcher is ready to run the study in the "laboratory" of the outside world. The traditional research view (Table 11) usually ignores the intentions of those researched and the details of their setting. As a result, researchers who postpone their contact with the phenomenon until completing their proposal almost always encounter problems which require at best revisions of their proposed research and at worst necessitate abandoning it altogether.

Planning applied research must occur in close and continuous contact with the potential participants and their setting. Margaret Patterson (1991), for example, exploring the topic of how veterinary students make the transition from academic work to their practicum, interviewed students about their experiences as well as their interest in participating in her study. In this way, she was getting in touch with the phenomenon.

Responsiveness (the second R), requires that researchers consider interviewees as resource people who can help them develop a workable proposal. This kind of interview is not akin to a "pilot study" in which the researcher tries out the final study in miniature; it is an acknowledgment that participants must be involved throughout the planning. Specifically, the researcher interviews potential participants using the Kolb Cycle interview to determine their attitudes to research and how this specific project might be meaningful. Potential participants are also interviewed to discover their experienced knowledge (implicit theories and images) on the topic.

When I began to use the New Three R's as an interview guide for doctoral researchers beginning their thesis work, I had not anticipated an additional benefit: that in becoming the first participants in their own research, described earlier, they would become more effective interviewers and better listeners. When researchers have brought out their own knowledge, they gain an awareness of their own position. Such awareness frees them to listen more openly:

> In being responsive to the stories of the women prisoners, I tried to define boundaries so that I would not confuse my own implicit theories with theirs. I sketched out a preliminary model of the process by which people break the law, but I couldn't allow this model to shape my responses. In my first few interviews, the importance of responding to what I heard from the women soon became evident. By weighing my implicit theories against what I heard from them, it became apparent to me that any one model would be inadequate in describing their experiences. Although this might seem obvious, it has been the practice of psychologists and sociologists in criminology to impose one model on all criminals.

Carrying out a responsiveness interview helps researchers proceed to Reciprocality, the third R or, as it was called earlier, the negotiation of intentions. Most researchers find that they first confront participants' intentions when they attempt to arrange an interview and find themselves reflecting on how to present their study to the participant. Having brought out their personal attitudes to research participation is the first step. They can then draw on their personal criteria of what would attract them personally to participate as a source of beginning the negotiation. These informal negotiations form the basis for the consent form which is a formal contract between participants and researcher.

6. Opening and remaining open to surprise in research

The challenge of trying to be aware of our own views in order to transcend them, if only briefly, is certainly not limited to the area of research. Piaget, for example, believed that young children begin life in a completely self-centered egocentric state but gradually grow out of their self-absorption. An alternative view is that most of us remain highly egocentric, but learn ways of disguising our self-absorption. Think about yourself and those who are close to you, and consider how many of us are capable of going beyond our own individual concerns.

A second example of our limited view is the concept of "assimilative projection" which describes the tendency to project one's characteristics, beliefs, and intentions onto others (i.e., everyone else must be like me). Again, think of your own experience, especially in relation to acknowledging and understanding those who are very different from yourself (the "opposite partners" exercises in Chapter One aims to overcome assimilative projection). A third example of the difficulty of transcending our biases comes from what Sarason calls axioms which are unexamined world views, or assumptions which guide us even though we are unaware of them. Examples of such axioms include the notions that education takes place in schools and that rationality will improve the human condition. Becoming aware of these axioms, let alone transcending them, is very demanding.

To be open to surprise, which is how I recast the challenge posed by "experimenter bias," researchers need to deal with their own egocentrism and their tendency to view others as being like themselves. They also need to become aware of their uninspected axioms and world views. This is a very large order.

Traditional research in human affairs proposes to meet the challenge (1) by eliminating or controlling such personal qualities of the researcher and (2) by making very logical and specific predictions which will either be confirmed or rejected by the evidence (hypothetico-deductive approach). This approach, which emulates the natural sciences, greatly reduces if not eliminates the practical value of research because it strips the researcher and the research of human relevance. The "grounded theory" approach proposed by Glaser and Strauss (1969) provides an alternative in that it views the research enterprise itself as a "tabula rasa" on which the researchers record the relevant aspects of the phenomena they are studying. It is interesting that although researchers who employ grounded theory are often viewed as completely opposite to those who work out of the tradition of logical positivism, they both recommend that researchers abandon their human qualities and personhood in the research enterprise.

I propose Research-as-renewal as a rapprochement which allows researchers to retain their personal qualities as allies, not as enemies. The question implicit in this approach is: How can the researcher be prevented from simply verifying his or her beliefs, that is, acting out a self-fulfilling prophesy in the negative sense? There is no simple answer, but a beginning is to suggest that at every stage, researchers be explicitly aware of their beliefs and intentions, and describe explicitly how they propose to remain open to surprise, that is, to disconfirmation or elaboration of their beliefs.

In selecting participants, researchers need to ask, Have I made an effort to find participants who are different from the other participants in the research and from myself? In designing the interview, the question is, Have I allowed an opportunity for, or indeed encouraged, participants to express views differing from my own? And in the analysis and interpretation of the material, researchers need to ask, To what extent have I explored alternative interpretations of the material? Sometimes researchers prepare hypothetical scenarios for alternative, unanticipated outcomes. I realize there is a contradiction in writing a scenario about what will surprise you, but at least researchers can ask the question, To what extent could the results/interpretation have been written without the inquiry?

One of the most innovative ways I have encountered of remaining open to surprise/dealing with bias is found in Susan Drake's study (1989) of teachers' use of visualization. She used the idea of subpersonalities as authoring different perspectives in her work which she needed to become aware of in order to transcend her own self-fulfilling prophecies as a researcher.

On Meeting My Biases

Spiritual Susan: There is a part of me that is intensely interested in spirituality. This is my favorite topic of conversation and I find myself attracted to individuals I consider to be spiritual or interested in the meaning and purpose of life. Unexpectedly, and to my delight, three of my participants were very spiritual people with whom I felt an identification. Spiritual Susan runs the risk of distorting this study by concentrating on the spiritual aspect and not seeing what is really there.

Successful Susan: This "I" is such a part of me that I really have trouble recognizing her. One of my committee members objected to my original questions because they smacked of my success orientation. I really couldn't see it. However, I dutifully deleted any questions which mentioned or implied success. Then I began to hear that bias from my participants. For example, a nursing educator had told me she used visualization to prevent colds. In one class session I was teaching I found out that she was hiding from me because she had a cold and didn't feel she'd been successful at visualization. Then my second participant said he didn't know if he was suitable for the study because his visualizations did not always work. I had to accept that I was communicating a success orientation to my participants. Since then, I believe that I was able to catch myself most of the time and that what I heard about is the actual experiences of the teachers in their lived experience.

Pro-Reflective Susan: A bias that I have come up against is that I really prefer reflective people. Some of my participants were more reflective than others. When interviewing a less reflective participant, my own bias could have influenced my attitude and jeopardized my interaction as a co-researcher. It could also blind me from hearing this experience as it was for the person. I had to be careful not to show impatience or probe further than the participant wished.

Salesperson Susan: I have spent many years selling visualization as a technique. It is hard for me to drop this role. For example, one of my participants is a novice in the use of this technique in the classroom but is very curious about learning more. After the first interview, I found myself offering her alternative ways to use it. During the interval between interviews she had tried my suggestions. This makes me more of a participant-observer than I was with my other participants. I have to be careful that in my salespersonship I don't contaminate my raw data. As well, I must constantly keep in mind that this study is an inquiry and not make extravagant claims for visualization.

Miss Thorough Susan: Miss Thorough wants to do a fine job on her thesis. (Shades of Successful Susan and Pro-Reflective Susan can be seen here.) As I proceeded in my data collection, I couldn't help but reflect and theorize. By the time I had collected two-thirds of my raw data, it occurred to me that a conceptual framework articulated by one of the participants seemed to fit all the data collected. Should I be hearing alarm bells? Would I force the remaining two cases into a framework that didn't really fit because I had preconceived ideas? (pp. 36–38)

Brader Brathwaite (1988) tackled the problem differently:

So it is at this point that I must begin to peel away the layers of hidden knowledge that I have acquired in my journey of life. This process of uncovering and bringing to the surface one's own personal theories relating to a phenomenon entails a great deal of risk that at the onset seems to outweigh any possible benefits. Those of us who decide to involve ourselves in this process and forge ahead to confront the hurdles of our own inner selves will take the largest leaps forward. (p. 26)

7. Researchers describe benefits and difficulties in Research-as-renewal

Finally, I present examples of the perceived benefits of this approach:

The most important benefit for me in this process was moving from the traditional perspective of a solo research effort to a collaborative, co-operative, and collegial approach. Through the interaction and sharing that took place, new relationships developed, deeper connections evolved, and belief and trust in ourselves and in one another were nurtured.

*   *   *

Arriving at a "place" where I could begin to write the research proposal has been as much a process of gaining self-knowledge as it has been of gaining knowledge about my research topic. The process included the use of imagery. After chasing a symbol of wisdom away (because it seemed to be pedestrian, uninspiring, and "not mine"), I experienced a feeling of well-being and a sense of clarity which validated my need to pursue my own implicit theories.

*   *   *

An extremely important aspect has been the extent to which my own ideas about research have been clarified and validated. I was able to articulate residual feelings which had not been thoroughly examined in a "hands-off" approach to research. Persons-in-relation and the New Three R's implicitly emphasize the process of doing research. Mainstream approaches to research emphasize "proving" and are by definition not amenable to movement. It is the movement or process of research which I find exciting, useful, and affirming.

* * *

The greatest benefit of this approach to my research has been the value I now place on experienced knowledge. This has led to a reflection on my own experienced knowledge and has resulted in an increased level of confidence and personal growth, a greater understanding and appreciation for research as a process of renewal, for both myself and those participating in my research.

* * *

The concept of beginning with ourselves and an Inside-out approach have influenced the paths I have chosen in my research journey. This approach was reaffirmed through a guided imagery session in class. When the "wiseperson" appeared without a gift, I was originally confused until I realized that the gift was within me. Throughout this journey, I would discover and re-discover this gift many times.

* * *

The imagery I experienced throughout the course has come to have great meaning for me. I have found this to be a wonderful source of energy. The transformation of the image of my work and my research, from a "bridge" to a "weaver," has had an influence on how I view the relationship between theory and practice within physical education. This image has encouraged me to reflect on my own undergraduate physical education.

* * *

The suggestion that my experienced knowledge was valuable and was a place to begin my research was reaffirming as well as useful in directing and organizing the future of my project.

Like anything worthwhile in life, Research-as-renewal requires persistence. The most frequently mentioned difficulty was for researchers to overcome their long-conditioned view about research as an objective, impersonalized venture to be recorded by a detached observer. The following comments illustrate this difficulty:

I had a difficult time overcoming the sense of threat from the traditional approach which is accepted and rewarded within the university community. As a result of these feelings, I found myself focusing on the negative images of my past experiences and my research. This became a blockage in my research journey which I had to overcome and in doing so I have not only opened up new developments in my research, but it has also helped me personally both to understand and to control the anger I had been experiencing. This type of research requires both self-reflection and an ability to communicate with others. These skills are not learned through reading or studying a statistics book; they require an investment of the self and a willingness to step down from the "high ground" of the "expert."

I found that in applying the Three R's my own underdeveloped modes of learning were being challenged. For example, I found that moving away from reflective observation to abstract conceptualization was somewhat difficult. I saw this as an opportunity to develop further my own developed and underdeveloped modes of learning.

Finally, I experienced some difficulty in overcoming a conditioned response to learning and the notion that the "answer" is out there. When I experienced blocks in my journey to date, my first reaction was to move outside to see what "research tells us." Initially, I had difficulty with imagery and therefore with the usefulness of it. But my willingness and persistence have paid off, as I have found this to be a great source of energy and guidance.

Despite this difficulty, many practitioners-turned-researchers find Research-as-renewal to be valuable, as indicated by the increasing number of doctoral theses completed in its spirit. Research-as-renewal also helps researchers confront the pragmatic reality that many face when they return to full-time jobs where they must negotiate time and energy to complete their thesis research. Unless the topic is close to their hearts and central to their values, it is unlikely that they will sustain the energy required to complete the project.

In this chapter, I have tried to raise your awareness about research in human affairs. Whether conducting research, or reading about it, inquiry plays a vital role in our lives especially as it is used to determine social and educational policy and decisions about practice. All of us need to be informed consumers of research reports, and I hope my attempts at demystification have set a foundation for developing such awareness. In contrast to traditional approaches, Research-as-renewal is liberating to both researcher and researched. It also opens the way for the future expression of human potential, releasing the flow of untapped and perhaps unimagined human resources within ourselves.

CHAPTER EIGHT

Renewing Ourselves: The Inner Journey

We shall not cease from exploration
And the end of all our exploring
Will be to arrive where we started
And know the place for the first time.

T. S. Eliot

People are increasingly hungry for self-knowledge to help them cope with problems in their daily lives. The signs of this hunger are evident in the proliferation of self-help books which promise the "quick fix" and the "one-minute solution." Pop psychology may provide temporary relief, but it is unlikely to set the foundation for sustained self-renewal. By contrast, self-help support groups, which are an example of sharing for self-renewal, embody the idea that expertise resides in ourselves and in those around us rather than in self-styled outside experts.

Like pop psychology, mainstream psychology is unhelpful, but for a different reason. In order to retain their power and control, experts in psychology and the other social sciences couch their knowledge in incomprehensible jargon — self-efficacy, attribution, internal control. In this chapter, I strive for a middle ground between the two psychologies, avoiding the quick fix on the one hand and jargon on the other as I develop the notion that renewing our lives is a continuous inner journey. I invite you to join me in this journey of self-renewal.

The essence of self-renewal is *movement*. This is illustrated by one of the first research studies conducted using George Kelly's theory, "A movement interpretation of threat" (Landfield, 1954). Specifically, the study identified persons who block our psychological movement by threatening us either by their example or by their expectations. Participants in the research began by bringing out their personal constructs — shy/assertive, creative/uncreative, open/closed to feelings. They then used their own personal rating scales to describe themselves in the past, in the present, and in the future. On some scales, the rating might be the same for all three, for example, fairly assertive in the past, the same now, and the wish to remain so. In such a case, there would be no movement. However, on other scales, participants might wish to move on a dimension, for example, rating oneself as closed to feelings in the past, somewhat more open now, and hoping to become more open in the future. This is a dimension of movement.

Landfield tested two predictions about how participants would experience others as threatening, and both were stated in relation to dimensions on which they were hoping to move, or in Kelly's terms, to "leave an old role behind." On those dimensions on which we hope to move (e.g., to become more open to our feelings), we will experience threats from two kinds of persons: those who *exemplify* the old role in themselves (i.e., are very closed to their feelings) and those who *expect* us to act according to the old role (i.e., remain closed to our feelings).

Landfield's study documents the process of stopping in our journey when what we really need to consider is how we can move along in our journey. So just as I reverse stingers, I reverse the underlying dynamic of Landfield's results. We can consider the dimensions on which we hope to move in a way that will facilitate our movement if we orient to others who (1) *exemplify* the new role (i.e., demonstrate openness to their feelings) or (2) expect us to act according to the quality we aspire to have in ourselves (i.e., display openness to feelings).

As you embark on your journey of self-renewal, I recommend that you review the qualities in the Spirit of Renewal framework (Table 7) because these qualities — respect, openness, optimism, patience, sense of humor, and most of all, faith — are essential for the journey of renewal.

This chapter is organized around your journey: the necessity of the trip, mapping the territory, what to do when you get lost, planning the journey, travel tips, avoiding roadblocks and detours, and traveling together.

Is This Trip Really Necessary?

Before embarking on an inner journey of renewal, you need to deal directly with the question, Why? Perhaps you are under great stress and need some way to cope with day-to-day pressures. Perhaps you would like to develop certain parts or qualities of yourself over the long run. Perhaps you have become interested in the ideas of the Spirit of Renewal and want to try to bring some of these beliefs into your life.

Whatever your intent, you will need to make a personal commitment to at least a brief time period on a regular basis. Like everything worthwhile in life, personal renewal is not a quick fix, and requires time and effort. At this point, many of you will be thinking, "But that's exactly my problem, I don't have *any* time for myself." In this case, the first question to deal with may be, How do I find the time to devote to my own renewal? Perhaps you have a very strict Critic who won't allow you to "indulge" in the luxury of self-reflection. Yet many people have found it possible to negotiate with their Critic to arrange for 30 minutes a day for themselves.

So the idea is to arrange a specific time for self-reflection every day and stick to it. If you are a night hawk, set aside time before going to bed for an evening review, or if you are a morning glory, take time just after rising. It is much like a commitment to a physical exercise regime which requires a goal, a will to carry it through, and a plan. Some people jog with a partner, and of course it is a little more difficult to conduct a morning review with someone else but you may choose to let another person know of your plan so that your commitment will be public. In any case, you must establish a commitment to work toward specific intentions during a specific period of time.

The basis of daily review is a journal or diary which will record your journey in terms of movement, obstacles, and so on, as discussed in the remaining sections of this chapter. You may never have kept a journal, you may even think, "But I'm not a reflective person, I'm action oriented. I can't sit in a chair for half an hour and just think about things." Maybe developing your underdeveloped reflective capacity needs to be your first goal. In addition, guides to journal keeping are available (e.g., *At a Journal Workshop,* Progoff, 1975).

Mapping Your Inner Territory and Resources

After making a commitment to renewing yourself, the next step is to map your inner territory by identifying your experienced knowledge (as described in Chapter One). This preliminary step is intended to both (1) identify the resources you have to draw on and (2) determine the area you wish to develop. Although I emphasized personal images to facilitate renewal, I re-introduce the other features of experienced knowledge — self-perception and implicit theories — because they, too, play a vital role in energy renewal.

Through identifying your own learning style, you will map your well-developed areas as well as your underdeveloped ones — for example, you may be a Northerner (p. 12) with an underdeveloped analytical capacity and this may define a direction for self-development and renewal. A second approach to self-perception is to identify some of your psychological dimensions and then assess yourself in terms of how you were in the past on this dimension, how you are now, and how you would like to be in the future as described in Landfield's study. To follow the Landfield approach to bring out your own dimensions, you may follow instructions in "How to Be Your Own Best Theorist" (Appendix 1 or Hunt, 1987) or adapt the REP test method in Appendix 5. In any case, bring out at least six or eight of your personal dimensions and rate yourself on each as you were in the past, as you are now, and as you would like to be. This enables you to identify "movement" dimensions (e.g., you might wish to become more assertive in future). Of course, you may simplify the procedure by simply asking yourself what characteristic or quality you would most like to develop. Either way you will have defined your goal for self-development.

Using the Kolb Cycle format to explore a positive professional experience is one way to bring out your *implicit theories*. Putting into words why you believe a positive experience occurred is a first step in expressing your implicit theory. As the examples of implicit theories in Appendix 2 show, implicit theories can also be succinctly expressed as stingers — for example, "Let the learner lead," "Self-esteem fosters knowledge; knowledge fosters self-esteem," or "Respect and expect." Readers wishing to express their implicit theories more fully as matching models may consult "How to Be Your Own Best Theorist" (Hunt 1980; Hunt 1987).

We should not forget *personal images* in identifying our resources. You may wish to personalize your journey image (for example, walking or flying), or perhaps you may wish to combine the journey with one of your images (for example, floating on a balloon or moving through musical passages).

When You Have Lost Your Way: Stress Management as Renewal

It is ironic that persons often in the greatest need of renewal, those who are nearly burnt out and are just getting by, see renewal as a luxurious option for those who have more time than they do. Viewed in terms of the Maslow hierarchy, they are at the survival level and they view renewal as something only for those seeking peak experiences. But renewal is very relevant for stress management "in the moment." From the energy renewal point of view, our experience of being "stressed out" is the same as being devoid of energy. So, for present purposes, stress management is viewed as maintaining or replenishing our energy. This is not to say the negative feelings associated with stress — feeling guilty, overwhelmed, or dispirited — are not significant personal experiences in and of themselves, but that they are often closely related to burnout and the depletion of personal energy.

One of the most frequently raised questions about the use of personal images is how they can serve one in the moment or, as one colleague put it, "in the heat of battle." How can I call on an image when there is very little time to go into it and draw from its energy? Although I did not emphasize it in Chapter Five, the management of stress is sometimes stated by colleagues as a concern to be dealt with in the C-RE-A-T-E Cycle: how can I cope with increasing demands and decreasing resources? In an example described earlier, Diane used her image of clearing a fog to cope with a staff conference she found stressful. The image served her "in the moment" to "clear the fog."

Each of us experiences stress in a distinctly personal way, so it is important to identify the situation and the nature of the stress we experience. How do you feel in the situation? What qualities do you need? Diane did not explicitly analyze the situation, but rather trusted the image of clearing the fog as a way to provide her with the mental, physical, and emotional state she needed to cope successfully with the situation.

Identifying your own experience of stress may require some reflection, but it is necessary. Individual experiences of stress vary widely and may hold elements, in different degrees, of anxiety, self-doubt, anger, rejection, envy, inadequacy, ignorance, shame, guilt, apathy, alienation, and confusion. You are likely to experience many of these feelings, but you should try to pin down the feelings which lead to your stress.

On the basis of your direct experience of stress, try to identify the quality you would need in the situation to alleviate these negative feelings. You may need confidence, patience, a capacity to focus, positive emphasis, clarity, or enthusiasm. As indicated in Chapter Five, you may access these qualities indirectly by calling on an image or more directly through accessing your own inner resources. An example of the use of imagery as a way to provide the quality indirectly is that of a colleague whose concern was her difficulty in communicating with groups. She took on the image of an eagle, which removed negative thoughts and cleared her mind, enabling her to proceed with positive action. This image worked without a detailed analysis of an action plan.

Several colleagues have expressed concern over losing control of their student/ clients and then feeling the stress of failure of responsibility. In such cases, colleagues frequently realize that they need help in "letting go" and in trusting their clients. One way to start is to look for images or perhaps parts of yourself which will help you access this quality. How can we find a part of ourselves capable of "letting go"? Most of us have been able to let go in one area of our life, and through identifying this area, we may build on this experience to do so in another area. This is similar to identifying a subpersonality within ourselves (Ferrucci, 1982) which possesses the desired qualities.

Sometimes people adopt a stinger to use "in the moment." For example, one colleague played a variation on the "Accentuate the positive" stinger: "Look for the beauty." Approaching a potentially stressful situation with these stingers shifts our emphasis, alters our perceptions, and finally alters our actions. When we take on new perspectives and try to adopt new actions, even new roles, these changes are likely to be greeted by puzzlement, if not suspicion, from others. Being stressed is often imbedded in the locked-in expectations of others (à la Landfield) which will not change easily, so be sure to keep your patience accessible.

Another example from researches comes from the colleague whose concern was with an excessively strict Critic which kept nagging her about her failure to move along on her thesis journey. She hit on an image of a tightrope walker carrying a balance rod, with her Critic on one side and her Creativity on the other. She went into the image, took one step at a time, crossed the rope successfully, then returned to do it again, each time feeling more confident. When asked what she was doing, she replied, "Looking ahead to where I'm going and taking one step at a time." In shifting emphasis to looking and to walking, she was no longer focused on the balancing rod which was now serving her general intention of moving along in her thesis by equalizing the voices of her Critic and her Creativity. She was no longer concerned with her Critic, which became a resource in the overall purpose.

One of the most valuable resources in managing stress is humor. I often use an imagery exercise developed to identify your image of fun and humor. Following is an image a student/colleague evoked:

> As you led us into the exercise I wondered if I would have an image: I often think that my sense of humor isn't well developed. This wonderful image came instantly.
> I was walking along the main street of a small town on the seashore and decided to go into the local theatre. I selected a seat in the middle of the theatre. The curtains separated and from the floor of the stage there emerged a full Dolphin Philharmonic Orchestra.
> They were delightful looking; each wearing a big smile and a colorful silk scarf. They played several pieces of happy music (I'm not able to name the music), and then the conductor turned to me in invitation: I had won the opportunity to conduct the orchestra. I walked to the stage and accepted the baton from the conductor and led the dolphins in a few frolicking pieces and returned to my seat.
> And then the most unexpected thing happened. The conductor turned to me again and sensed that I wanted more. She bowed deeply and pointed her baton at me: I immediately did a great dolphin leap to the stage and began again to conduct this wonderful orchestra.
> This was a great experience, unexpected and wonderfully funny.

The image of the Dolphin Philharmonic Orchestra was so delightful that not only did she herself continue to use it when she was under stress, but several others in the class acknowledged that they too found it a valuable way to release their uneasiness in the stress of the moment. Bringing out your own image of humor can be a very valuable resource to use "in the moment." Another colleague's image of humor involved people riding bumper cars at a carnival, an image which he used to view heated interactions. The image provided the needed shift in perspective and hence a relief from strain which helped him cope with otherwise stressful situations. In relation to overwhelming stress, these examples may seem trivial, but yet you need to try one or, better, create your own.

While you need to have immediate, short-term strategies for stress management, you also need to have long-term initiatives for your journey of self-development. In the next section I discuss planning your trip (deciding on your intentions of self-development and renewal) and then I offer some travel tips for your journey.

Planning and Preparing for Your Trip

Where to? Selecting your destination. In mapping your inner territory, you may have identified a particular journey you would like to make. One of the most likely long-term inner journeys is that of developing your underdeveloped learning style. As I mentioned in *Beginning with Ourselves*, I have been spending the past several years attempting to develop my "Northern" mode, that is, my openness to my feelings and the feedback they provide.

Also, you might identify a dimension (e.g., assertiveness or creativity) on which you are hoping to move, through assessing yourself on this dimension in past, present, and future relationships. Or, closely related, you may wish to get in touch with a quality to which you aspire (e.g., patience, enthusiasm, or authenticity). Finally, you may wish to develop one or more of the values in the Spirit of Renewal framework (e.g., synergy of sharing, positive emphasis). This is similar to moving toward a desired quality and, in both cases, a long-term journey.

Before embarking on your journey, you will need to reflect on why you want to travel and what provisions and resources you will need along the way. Considering why you want to develop in this direction is essential because your persistence and perseverance will be tested along the way, and if you are not committed to staying the course, you will not be likely to reach your destination.

The next step in planning is to review the destination as specifically as possible as well as your provisions (resources) for moving along. For example, let us imagine you have chosen to develop more patience.

1. What is the experience of patience like for you? How does it feel? What is your body like when you are patient? What are your thoughts when you are patient?
2. Does the quality have a related image, that is, what is your personal image of

patience? Related to this, what does it look like, sound like, smell, taste, and feel like?

3. Review your earlier experiences with the quality. In what situations have you displayed patience? Is there a part of yourself (a subpersonality) which exemplifies patience? How can you call this part on stage?
4. How can you identify/sense patience in others? What outstanding examples of patience have you observed directly or sensed indirectly in books, films, tapes? What person best exemplifies this quality?
5. What are the personal obstacles to developing the quality? What interferes with your displaying patience and how can you overcome this?

Travel Tips

Now that you are packed and your itinerary is mapped out, you are ready to travel. Remember that you need to chart your journey through your daily review, reflecting on how far you have travelled, road blocks encountered, and plans for the next day's journey.

1. Make an effort to interact with persons *who exemplify* the quality you aspire to, that is, people who show patience, as suggested at the beginning of the chapter. If appropriate, you might discuss with others how the quality is brought into action.
2. Make an effort to interact with persons who *expect* you to display the quality — persons who expect you to be patient. This provides an opportunity to try out the new quality in a supporting situation. It is equally important to avoid initially trying it out with persons who will threaten you by expecting the opposite, locking you into your old, unsatisfying role.
3. Try displaying the quality in new situations — for example, try out the quality of patience in a situation where others have no preconceived impression of you or any expectations of how you will react. This suggestion comes from George Kelly's (1955) advice to try on a new role in non-threatening situation so that you can see how it feels.
4. If possible, seek feedback from others when you have been attempting to display this quality. How did they perceive you? Patient or impatient? Did they find your actions appropriate?
5. In reviewing your efforts to develop the quality, attempt to identify your inner state when you were successful at expressing it, that is, try to raise your awareness of bringing out the quality so that you gain control over its use.

6. As time goes by, reflect on how this new quality fits with your other qualities/beliefs. Spend some time reflecting on how patience is becoming integrated with your other qualities. This is in the spirit of psychosynthesis which proposes the integration of subpersonalities/qualities (e.g., Ferrucci, 1982).

7. As will be discussed in the section "Traveling Together," you may wish to work on your self-development with a partner who can help you reflect on your actions.

Dealing with Roadblocks: Outside Experts and Other Barriers to Renewal

Bring back your Critic from its vacation, or wherever you sent it, so it is ready to confront those who claim to be experts in human affairs. Our culture tends to rely on outside experts as a primary source of knowledge, yet as I have argued in almost every page of this book, these experts usually know no more than most other people, and sometimes less, when we take a critical look at how they know what they know and compare it with our own experienced knowledge.

Why do we need to demystify the outside experts? We may save some money by not paying their fees and by not buying their books, but a more important reason is that excessive reliance on experts cuts us off from our own experienced knowledge and ultimately from our own sources of energy. When we are forced to rely on experts, we usually remain mystified, powerless, and lacking in confidence about our own knowledge and our own good sense to guide our actions.

Therefore, I propose a set of questions intended as a credibility checklist for outside experts. It is primarily for teachers to use when they encounter an expert brought in for their professional development, but I think it may be appropriate in other areas, for example, psychotherapy and counselling. You ask the expert:

1. Where do you believe that knowledge about human affairs comes from? Personal experience, theories, research, or some other source? Can you give an example of why you believe this?

2. What is your own personal/professional experience that qualifies you to be an expert in human affairs?

3. How do you propose to find out what we already know so that you learn from us as well as adapt your communication about your knowledge?

4. What tools can you offer us to learn more about ourselves and our practice so that we can share it with each other?

5. How can you help us create a climate in which our experienced knowledge and untapped resources can flow freely?

6. Finally, and most important, how do you propose to work with us so that we can be self-sufficient, and will no longer need your expertise?

"Research tells us. . . ." How often have you come across this phrase or its equivalent? "Research tells us that personal health worsens as you grow older." "Research tells us that poor people have fewer opportunities." These cliches are designed to get your attention so that you can consider why it is that our culture requires "Research to tell us" what we already know from our experience? Isn't it likely that its implicit purpose is to sustain the power and control of the outside experts and to restrict our own sense of knowing about human affairs?

As discussed in the previous chapter, we need to be especially vigilant in considering research purporting to show the effects of such things as day care, controlled drinking, or physical exercise because in complex areas of this sort, we often encounter contradictory findings or hear one story at one time and another with a complete opposite point of view a few years later. There is also the version of "Research tells us . . ." from the opinion surveys. These cases require a critical approach more complex than that suggesting the six questions I have listed for the outside experts, but perhaps I can suggest a few ways to begin.

First, when you read research about human affairs, always compare it to your own experience, and if possible, ask others about it as well. Second, try to find out who the participants in the research were and why they participated (as described in the previous chapter), especially why they would want to provide information. Third, try to identify the vested interests or implicit values of those conducting the research to determine whether the research reflects a self-fulfilling prophesy or has a been designed to be open to surprise. In short, try to dig beneath the anonymity of "Research tells us . . ." to use your Critic. This is important, for I am convinced that in conducting research into human affairs, it is possible to find exactly opposite results simply by selecting different participants and using different methods. (Perhaps this is the most cynical statement I have made in this book.)

Like it or not, we live in the Age of Information where we are flooded by Information-as-knowledge . . . data . . . data . . . data. This flood of information not only overloads us, but it also cuts us off from our own knowing and our own sources for energy renewal. We need to raise questions about the nature of Information-as-knowledge so that we can base our foundation on Knowledge-as-process and Knowledge-as-experience. In so doing, we will also need to deal with the occasional issue on which Knowledge is pitted against Experience, for example, in the reconstruction of history. Historians may gain knowledge about the past through studying archival material. Occasionally, someone who was there will disagree with their findings so that the line is drawn between experience and knowledge. These two sources of understanding are fused in our experienced knowledge. And this needs to be our base for considering the flood of information we encounter.

We also live in the Age of Computers. Computers can be enormously valuable, of course, but there must be a limit to the claims that many computer scientists make regarding artificial intelligence and the replacement of human beings. Despite claims to the contrary, human beings can never be completely replaced by computers. Indeed, the distinguishing feature of persons rendering human services is that they can do what computers cannot and never will be able to do, namely, respond to unanticipated situations with their heads, hearts, and bodies. I should make it clear that I am not recommending we ignore computers and the search for artificial intelligence. Rather, I'm suggesting that through connecting with our human potential, we will feel affirmed that the human condition is unique and cannot be replaced by a machine, although the achievement of human potential can, of course, be facilitated greatly by such machines.

Traveling Together

Traveling together whether with a partner or in a group involves the qualities of sharing as co-creation — good will, non-judgmental orientation, respect, openness to feelings, and trust. Perhaps the best example of traveling together and the equity of expertise is the enormous increase of self-help support groups which are estimated to involve at this time over 15 million people in North America. These groups represent respect for the experience of group members rather than the impersonal advice of outside experts.

Whether formal or informal, these support groups often epitomize the Spirit of Renewal with respect to all five of its beliefs, beginning with the equity of expertise. In fact, many support groups have developed when prospective members came to realize that outside experts did not have many answers. Members believe specifically that persons who have had common experiences, whether these consist in living with a relative who is terminally ill, dealing with an addiction, or dealing with a handicap, possess experienced knowledge which can be of practical value. Most support groups exemplify the synergy of sharing in their discussions, with special emphasis on the emotional support that derives from sharing experiences and experienced knowledge.

In my experience as a facilitator of support groups, I find that the notion of positive emphasis is equally important. Pooling experienced knowledge from positive experiences provides a rich source of knowledge for addressing concerns. For example, as a person with limited vision, I work in a support group with other visually handicapped persons. When we address a common concern, for example, how to deal with the reaction of people who think we have snubbed them because we have not recognized them, we each reflect on a positive experience in dealing with this problem. We consider, perhaps, why it worked and pool our experienced knowledge on the topic to derive some guides for action. My experience with this group has also showed me that outside experts can contribute when they meet the credibility checklist in the preceding section. In this case, the outside expert is an optometrist who occasionally meets with us; he has a remarkable sensitivity for each person's visual world and also believes firmly in helping us to become as independent and self-affirming as possible.

As discussed in Chapter Seven, doctoral students often find that forming thesis support groups can be very helpful. In this case, I have specifically facilitated C-RE-A-T-E Cycle groups for students to pool their resources, receive emotional support, and gain direction for moving along on their thesis journey.

While the equity of expertise and synergy of sharing provide the basic direction for support groups, they are fuelled by a positive emphasis and a sense of humor. These ingredients are essential to developing the nurturing and sustaining climate which is one of their secrets. As I wrote this sentence, I realized that I was identifying a belief I once expressed about support groups. Because they approach them from Outside-in, experts have never been able to figure out why support groups such as AA work. I do not pretend to understand their power completely, but I am sure it begins with locating the expertise *within* the group and its members, a shift in location which is very threatening to outside experts.

Gentle as You Go

In conclusion, I propose that we add another quality to those in the Spirit of Renewal — gentleness. I emphasize this quality because I have come to realize how important it is to be gentle with ourselves on our journeys of renewal. Being gentle with others is also highly recommended, but what we often neglect is the need to be gentle with ourselves.

Let me end with an example. A few years ago, at the conclusion of one of my Learning Styles classes, my students presented me with an Inside-out T-shirt. It not only carried the literal message, INSIDE OUT, but the shirt itself was inside-out so that the printing was on the "wrong" side (something which bothered my grandchildren when I wore it — "Grandpa, your shirt's inside out.") It was not until sometime later that I realized the significance or the double meaning of the Inside-out shirt: going Inside-out means turning yourself Inside-out, exposing yourself in new ways. (Think about what it would be like to have your skin turned Inside-out.) This image brought out for me the vulnerability we experience as we begin our journeys of renewal. Perhaps, for a time, we are without our protective armor; we are prickly, sensitive, uncertain, and we need, above all things, gentle treatment. So it is in this spirit that I wish you well on your journey of renewal. May it be exciting, mysterious, affirming, full of surprises, and fun. Gentle as you go!

APPENDIX 1

Guided Imagery Instructions

Note: I suggest that you personalize the instructions below by reading them into a tape recorder. They are appropriate for evoking images from any kind of positive experience, but I suggest you begin with a positive professional experience as in the exercise at the beginning of Chapter Three. Once you have identified the experience, you are ready to begin. Remember, you will be in control during the exercises: if anything happens that you do not like or do not want to deal with, just tell it to go away.

Put down any materials you may have been using: pen, book, or whatever, and make yourself comfortable and close your eyes. We will first take a few moments to prepare ourselves by breathing deeply, relaxing, and clearing our minds. . . . Let's begin by paying attention to breathing. . . . Breathe deeply . . . noticing your breathing, which we usually take for granted. . . . As you are letting out your breath, allow yourself to relax, first in your legs, allowing the tension to float away so that you feel more relaxed . . . breathing deeply . . . as you allow your back and neck to relax, and the tension eases out through your arms so that your shoulders and back feel more relaxed. . . . Breathing . . . relaxing . . . now allow those ideas and thoughts in your mind to fade away so that your mind is uncluttered . . . you may reclaim these later, but for now allow your mind to become clear, to go in directions you wish . . . breathing deeply, and as you do allow your stomach and chest to relax, the tensions floating away so that your entire body feels relaxed and in tune . . . breathing . . . relaxing . . . clearing. . . . If doubts or questions pop into your head just send them away, and allow yourself this time for yourself, a time to be with yourself, a time just to be . . . patience fills you. Breathing . . . relaxing, and clearing.

Now, recall that positive professional experience as completely as possible. Begin with the setting where it occurred, then the time . . . time of year . . . the weather, time of day. Next put yourself into that situation as it happened along with the other people who were there. Make sure you are *in* the scene, not observing it. . . . Before beginning to re-live the experience, open yourself to all of the sense experiences of the situation . . . what it looked like, the sounds, the smells, the touches, and especially your feelings. As you re-experience the situation, try to open yourself to your feelings of that moment as fully as possible, and allow those feelings to develop as they will . . . now for a few moments, go back into that experience and re-live it as it happened as fully and completely as possible. If you find yourself distracted, focus on your feelings. . . . Go ahead . . . focus on your feelings. Take a few moments to go through the experience.

[Leave 30-40 seconds blank on tape for reliving the experience]

Now it's time to let the experience go. Allow the parts of the experience to fade away, but hold onto your feelings in the moment so that they are very much with you. Allow the experience gradually to fade while you retain your feelings. . . . Patience . . . now, opening yourself as much as possible to what may happen, you find that an image will present itself. It may come in any form. Don't force it, just open yourself and notice what happens. The image may be through sounds or it may be an intensification of your feelings . . . however it presents itself, allow it to develop and become what it wants to be. . . . Patient and open . . . no rushing. . . . As the image develops, open yourself to any communication from the image. . . . Make yourself comfortable with your image, perhaps by dialoguing with it, this is quite possible in imagery. . . . If nothing has happened, be patient, relaxed and open for what may happen. Don't force it. . . .

Once you are comfortable with your image, take a few moments to enter into it, to become the image. If you need to re-arrange anything so that you can live in the image for a few moments, make these changes, then enter into your image. What is this like? How do things look? Sound? Especially, how does it feel, being your image? Is there a special quality which comes to you as you are your image? As you are experiencing your image from inside, you are aware of your connecting with part of yourself and you feel good about that. Now come back out of the image and express your thanks for this connection. Your image, in turn, presents you with a token, a symbol which you may use in future if you wish to connect with it again. You accept with thanks.

For the next few moments, allow yourself just to be with your image, no questions, no worries about what it means, just relax and be there for a few moments (15 to 20 seconds blank on tape). Now, before the image fades away, consider what is the quality you are experiencing, allow yourself to become keenly aware of that quality.

Now it's time for the image to fade away . . . to leave in whatever form it came while you are left with your feelings and the quality which the image brought out in you. You sit quietly for a few moments allowing the experience to sink in, especially your feelings about this new-found resource with which you have connected.

Now it's time for you to come back very gradually . . . first pay attention to your breathing again . . . still feeling quite relaxed, you are feeling good about the experience . . . even if very little happened or it was not what you had expected, you realize that connecting with your imagination takes time and patience, and you have made an important first step. Whatever happened, you feel you have made a beginning. You realize that making the connection needs patience, openness, and being gentle with yourself. Filled with these thoughts, you gradually become aware of your physical presence back in the room. Your feet on the floor, your being seated in the chair . . . when you are ready open your eyes, look around, take a stretch, and allow yourself to become adapted to being back in the room. Take a few moments to jot down any notes you wish to make about the experience.

APPENDIX 2

Experienced Knowledge Summaries

A.

Self-Perception

Without any doubt, I am a Northerner. How often have I told people that I am a doer, not a thinker. Well, it is time for me to dwell on AC — abstract conceptualization. Small groups, hands-on activities, summarizing the text or my notes are the ways in which I learn most confidently. I continue to find difficulties listening to a lecture or tapes.

Implicit Theories

The stinger which best serves my style is "Risk-taking promotes growth." Believe in yourself and don't be afraid to get involved, make change, and do your best. The positive experiences on which I have focused during these exercises occurred because I believe in others and in myself. One lesson which I learned years ago was to use the talents and gifts of the staff members wherever I was to work. I have found that when I believe in them, they in turn believe in me, and we trust each other. In a trusting climate, we can accomplish more than most dream.

Personal Images

A fugue written for woodwinds and percussion. The melody was "Variation of a Theme," that of the Happy Birthday tune. This came to mind perhaps because we were reflecting on a positive experience which was for me a celebration of the arts.
    The subject was a solo bassoon, while the first answer was the clarinet. This fugue was written for four voices and the subject represented me while the answers represented the children with whom I was working; the audience for whom we performed and the organizers of this gala event. Rarely did the bassoon refrain from playing, although at times it was very much in the background. The light, lively flutes were those energy-filled children (the younger singers), while the timpani and tambourines were the grade 8 boys; the voices of the seniors in charge were from

the clarinet family — strong and ever so sure of themselves. The oboes, in harmony with the entire section represented the enthusiastic audience. The last solo subject was myself, alone on the bus, after the performances were completed and the children were home.

B.

Self-Perception

- Southerner — highest on abstract conceptual
- Very undeveloped CE — tend to intellectualize & rationalize
- Constantly want to know "why"
- Want to know why "image" developed and can't get rid of the "critic" and go with the image
- Enjoy new ideas, interaction, discussion and challenge

Implicit Theories

- Choice, not chance, determines destiny
- Individuals have the power within them to be what they want to be
- Individuals need success and a good self-concept develops through understanding and believing in oneself
- Children, young adults and seniors can all learn/develop the skills required for successful communication in the "world"
- Each person should strive for increased knowledge/awareness/learning throughout their lifetime
- Each person is unique and it is that uniqueness that gives society its strength

Images of Teaching

- Snow White-like figure — perhaps mother earth/nature?
- Environment — the woods — rich, lush, natural, interrelated
  all resources are already there
  warm sun sparkling on pond
  a happy place
- Animals all around Snow White — playing, talking, laughing
  interactive environment
  animals in little groups — go off and work together, listen to Snow White who seems to be a wise story teller
- not dependent on Snow White — have resources and ability to learn from other animals

C.

Self-Perception

- Westerner
- Active experimentation
- I would rather "play with something"
- I don't generally read directions until I get "stuck" but usually through working with something I meet with success
- Underdeveloped RO, usually want to "dive right in"
- Impatient

Implicit Theories

- Knowing yourself is the first step towards liking yourself
- Learning *should* and *can* be exciting and fun
- Success and responsibility for success are great motivators
- Anything can be accomplished if broken into small enough parts
- Being direct and consistent is important
- If a student is interested and motivated, other problems diminish
- Success in peer-related work enhances self-confidence

Personal Images

- Standing on a high cliff, cool air (smells like fall, autumn) feeling I can and will be able to jump off and fly
- Feeling free, uninhibited, able to explore, swoop
- Smelling air that is like autumn probably doesn't relate to feelings of returning to school but rather the fresh, clear, newness of it. It is one of, on further reflection, returning to school gives me those expectant faces. A very exciting time.
- Perhaps the flying or free falling is related to immersing myself in a new year.

D.

Self-perception

I tend to be analytical and evaluate situations. I am adept at drawing parallels and synthesizing information. I enjoy thinking. I found it interesting to consider that my skills might be of benefit in research and planning departments. I like to challenge existing ideas and my students tell me I am always asking "why?" I find it easier to rationalize an experience and make alterations for the future than to recall specific details from the event.

Implicit Theories

"Chance Favors a Prepared Mind"
I need to have a challenge in my life. I have found that these challenges, while sometimes threatening, become opportunities for undreamed-of possibilities. Each opportunity builds my confidence and opens new doors. Opportunities are an indication of my awareness levels on receptivity to new options. If, in fact, I seize the opportunity and take the risk, I must have subconsciously been prepared for the adventure. My implicit theory is a realization of my potential and a rationalization of the risk.
"The gods cannot help those don't seize the opportunity."

Personal Images

I imagine that I am at a birthday party. There is laughter, there is fun. We are all very special because we are at the party. There are games and prizes, followed by a cake and favors. Those are the planned events, but it is more often the unexpected that remains forever in our memory. I never imaged that there would be a time without another birthday party.

I imagine that I am up at bat. I cannot predict the pitch or my timing. I need to hit the ball for my team and, more honestly, for myself. If only I can get to first, then there is a chance to make it home. My uniform is an important part of my identity. It makes me feel and speak like a real baseball player.

APPENDIX 3

Images of Change

Note: As you consider these and the following lists of images, try them out for yourself, don't evaluate them from outside. Associated feelings are in brackets.

1. Locomotive with direction and clarity (good; today I'm lacking direction).
2. Circles coming from a core — non-random (anxiety — long time to g(r)o(w).
3. Isolated on a desert island, aware of ocean (peace, freedom, liberation).
4. Large mouth open wide, screaming, then becomes less wide open, singing pleasantly (fear of loss of control).
5. Series of circles . . . yellow, warm, confident . . . wearing down a rocky shore of fear and inhibition (mixed: fear and happy expectation).
6. Beautiful ordinary red rose . . . not trying to be anything else . . . thorns (whole, alive, and in the moment).
7. Victory sign . . . cheer of winning . . . fist held high (comforting).
8. Out of the cold ashes of yesterday, a phoenix rises through a pall of smoke unfamiliar like a new style of clothing . . . flying above the clouds.
9. Waves constantly in motion with ups and downs . . . potential for storm. . . power (good).
10. Cycle process like moon in relation to sun (frightening and exciting).
11. Organic image of cocoon which contains elements and timing of change. Only a skilled biologist can predict the nature of a butterfly (excitement mixed with anxiety).
12. Skating in game of shinny . . . on defense so must move quickly . . . both resist and initiate (terrific . . . concentrated, able, a bit under threat).
13. Flying spiritually . . . flying in a space as I did in a dream (great, challenging, exhilarating).
14. Skiing near goats in the mountains . . . gliding smoothly most of the time (absorbed, free spirit, but facing new challenges).
15. Sunflower growing with other plants in garden . . . plants twisting and winding (breakthrough, freedom, excitement).
16. An eggshell on the river floating down (excitement and anticipation).

APPENDIX 4

Other Images

Kit's Image

I see myself as a bright, colorful, transparent bubble that floats above a flock of Canada geese who are making their path toward the small lake. This bubble is alive and radiant because I see myself as an outgoing, friendly person. As I float in the air, I pulse in and out, I jump high, I wrap myself around my colleagues (the geese).

As time passes, the bubble bursts forth and starts exploding into millions of bubbles. As the bubble transforms its shape, it jumps higher with energy. It begins to wrap itself around the geese, touching and interacting with the flock. Sensing new confidence, direction, and acceptance, the bubble is now having more fun interacting with the flock. However, the bubble knows that it needs time to rest, observe, listen, and reflect, even though the bubble enjoys action almost immediately. The exploration and experimentation continues. There is a sense of "one," sharing new ideas and building positive attitudes.

After the guided imagery experience, I wanted to draw my images. At first, I tried to avoid writing poetry, but after my drawing session, I felt more confident.

> **A Summary of my Image**
> A transparent, colorful
> bubble floating,
> exploding, changing shape,
> journeying up and down,
> exploring, touching someone

It is a journey of self-discovery and adventure. I like to think that the bubble never breaks — it bursts into more bubbles, and it interacts with the wonderful living creatures, the Canada geese. For me, the Canada geese symbolize the idea of hope for the future. The peaceful, elegant birds strive to maintain their existence in our lakes. They always look so grand, peaceful and relaxed as they glide smoothly through the water. My vision of the geese is always clear as they are one of my favorite sights.

Many feelings envelop me when I am in this relaxed state of mind. I am at peace with myself: I feel a sense of warmth and comfort. I feel that I am being energized. I am sensitive to my environment.

My image needs a kaleidoscope of color to keep it floating and changing shape. I like my image very much. As a child, I always remember blowing bubbles and chasing them in the garden. It is like reliving a fantasy world, a world viewed through a child's eyes. I tend to be a sensitive and nostalgic person.

Images of Practice
(Associated Qualities)

1. Stained glass window . . . Sun streaming through me reflecting beautiful colors. (Good will)
2. I am a shepherd travelling across a fragrant valley with my flock. (Sensitivity)
3. I am the ocean. The deep and mysterious aspect of the ocean intrigues me. I am very powerful and important. (Power)
4. Raft. Supportive, adaptable, soft, yet firm enough, floats freely, comfortable, mobile, protective, drown-proof.
5. As a sunflower, I radiate warmth, confidence, and enthusiasm. I stand erect and tall. I draw seeds (my students) to me through my bright yellow petals which represent my vibrance and humor. The seeds eventually burst and fall in various types of soil. Some will germinate immediately, others will lie dormant. (Warmth)
6. A simmering cup of tea that has steeped for the appropriate time. (Patience)
7. A hot air balloon with birds landing and taking off (students) — brightly colored and untethered, in the company of a lot of other balloons. (Peace, Freedom)
8. My favorite image is that of a migrating beaver building a new dam and pond. (Warmth, Nurturing)

Images of Collaboration

Collaborative research is like . . . an octopus — "tentacles" reaching for sustenance — sharing and/or ingesting — and reaching out again.

*   a jigsaw puzzle with people coming together to formulate a whole picture
*   serious dating, hopefully leading to full-scale romance
*   a partnership of the dance of ballet
*   a college mixer, early in the fall of the year
*   a team of unmatched horses pulling together
*   baking a cake . . . hoping that the ingredients are going to produce what you think you want
*   carpenters working together to construct a building
*   farming — planting the seed, working it, fertilizing it, praying and waiting until harvest

APPENDIX 5

Bringing Out Your Concepts of Interpersonal Relationships

This exercise is based on the Role Construct Repertory Test (Hunt, 1987, pp.164-171), and allows you to identify your concepts or dimensions through sorting cards. In this case, you need six 3 x 5 cards or small pieces of paper. Number the cards in the upper right hand corner from 1 to 6. On each card write your name and the name of another person with whom you have a relationship. The pairs may be from your work, such as yourself and one of your students/clients, or you may write down pairs in which you and the other person are not in your work setting, you and your spouse or important other, you and a friend, etc. Make sure that in each case, you and the other person know each other well enough that you can form an impression about the relationship.

Now, select cards, 1, 2, and 3. Which two of these are alike in terms of the relationship? When you have made your selection, answer the question, "How are they alike in terms of the relationship, that is, how would I describe the relationship?" Follow the same procedure for cards 4, 5, and 6, recording your description of how the relationship is similar. Then go on to cards 1, 3, and 5, then cards 2, 4, and 6 so that you wind up with four *different* descriptions of interpersonal relations. Complete the form below by recording the four characteristics and their opposites so you have created four dimensions.

Response Form for Interpersonal Dimensions

Characteristics		Opposite
(1, 2, 3)	_____	_____
(4, 5, 6)	_____	_____
(1, 3, 6)	_____	_____
(2, 4, 6)	_____	_____

These are your personalized dimensions for viewing your relations with others. You may compare them with the dimensions in Chapter Four and also consider how you might use them to change a relationship as in the "Movement" dimensions in Chapter Eight.

APPENDIX 6

C-RE-A-T-E Cycle

Form for C-RE-A-T-E Cycle

1. Concern: I would like to . . .

2. REflect: The image I would like to apply is that of . . .

3. Action plan: Applying the image to my concerns, I develop the following plan of action . . .

    "green lights"

4. Try out: When?

5. Experience: How did it go? What are the next steps?

REFERENCES

Abbey, D. S., Hunt, D. E., and Weiser, J. C. (1985). Variations on a theme by Kolb: A new perspective for understanding counselling and supervision. *The Counselling Psychologist*, 13, 477-501.

Assagioli, R. (1965). *Psychosynthesis.* New York: Viking.

Bandler, R., and Grinder, J. (1979). *Frogs into princes.* Moab, Utah: Real People Press.

Beattie, M. (1991). *Teacher learning and inquiry as curriculum development.* Unpublished doctoral dissertation thesis in progress. University of Toronto (OISE).

Belenky, M. F., Clinchy, B. M., Goldberger, N. R., and Tarule J. M. (1986). *Women's ways of knowing.* New York: Basic Books.

Bernstein, B. (1979). *Action, relation, and transformation: A study of Viola Spolin's Theater Games.* Unpublished doctoral dissertation. University of Toronto (OISE).

Bolin, F., and Falk, J. M. (Eds.) (1987). *Teacher renewal.* New York: Teachers College Press.

Berman, P., and McLaughlin, M. W. (1978). *Federal programs supporting educational change, Vol. VIII: Implementing and sustaining innovations.* Santa Monica, CA: The Rand Corporation.

Brackman, T. (1976). Experiential Knowledge: A new concept for the analysis of self-help groups. *Social Science Review.* 445-456.

Brathwaite, B. (1988). *Teachers as persons, practitioners and theorists.* Unpublished doctoral dissertation. University of Toronto (OISE).

Bray, S. (1986). *Exploring the instructional process in a professional school: A study of instructors' thinking.* Unpublished doctoral dissertation. University of Toronto (OISE).

Cole, A. (1987). *Teachers' spontaneous adaptation: A mutual interpretation.* Unpublished doctoral dissertation. University of Toronto (OISE).

Connelly, F. M., and Clandinen, D. J. (1988).*Teachers as curriculum planners.* New York/Toronto: Teachers College Press/OISE Press.

Drake, S. (1989). *An exploration of teachers' experience with visualization in their lives and in their classrooms.* Unpublished doctoral dissertation. University of Toronto (OISE).

Eisner, E. W. (1991). *The enlightened eye.* New York: Macmillan.

Ferrucci, P. (1982). *What we may be.* Los Angeles: Jeremy P. Tarohar.

Fox, D. (1983). Personal theories of reading. *Studies in Higher Education,* 8, 151-163.

Gardner, J. W. (1982). *Self-renewal.* New York: Norton.

Glaser, B. G., and Strauss, A. L. (1967). *The discovery of grounded theory.* Columbus: Aldine Publishing.

Grimett, P. P., and Erickson, G. L. (Eds.) (1988). *Reflection in teacher education.* Vancouver/New York: Pacific Educational Press/Teachers College Press.

Heider, F. (1958). *The psychology of interpersonal relations.* New York: Wiley.

Hunt, D. E. (1976). Teachers are psychologists, too: On the application of psychology to education. *Canadian Psychological Review,* 17, 210-218.

Hunt, D. E. (1978). Theorists are persons, too. In C. Parker (Ed.) *Encouraging student development in college.* Minneapolis: University of Minnesota Press.

Hunt, D. E. (1980). How to be your own best theorist. *Theory Into Practice,* 19, 287-293.

Hunt, D. E. (1987). *Beginning with ourselves.* Cambridge, MA/Toronto: Brookline Books/OISE Press.

Hunt, D. E. (1989). Teacher Centres: Professional renewal for the nineties, *Orbit,* 20, 4.

Hunt, D. E. (1990). Person, culture, and the initiation of change: comments on D. Britzman's review of *Beginning with ourselves. Curriculum Inquiry,* 20, 75-78.

Ingalls, J. D. (1975). *Human energy.* New York: Learning Concepts.

Kelly, G. A. (1955). *The psychology of personal constructs.* New York: Norton.

Kluckhohn, C., and Murray, H. (Ed.) (1948). *Personality in nature, society, and culture.* New York: Knopf.

Kolb, D. A. (1975). Toward an applied theory of experiential learning. In C. Cooper (Ed.), *Studies of group process.* (pp. 33-57). New York: Wiley.

Kolb, D. A. (1984). *Experiential learning.* Englewood Cliffs, NJ: Prentice-Hall.

Landfield, A. W. (1954). A movement interpretation of threat. *Journal of Abnormal and Social Psychology,* 49, 529-532.

Lewin, K. (1951). *Field theory in social science.* New York: Harper Torchbooks.

Little, J. W. (1984). Seductive images and organizational realities in professional development. *Teachers College Record,* 86, 84-102.

MacMurray, J. (1961). Persons in relation. London: Farber & Farber.

Morgan, G. (1986). *Images of organization.* Newbury Park, CA: Sage.

Morgan, G. (1989). Keynote address to Ontario Society for Training and Development, Toronto, Ontario, November 13.

Mumby, H. (1985). Teachers' professional knowledge: A study of metaphor. Paper presented at AERA.

Patterson, M. (1991). *A study of the externship experience of veterinary students.* Unpublished doctoral dissertation. University of Toronto. (OISE)

Polanyi, M. (1962). *Personal Knowledge.* New York: Harper Row.

Progoff, I. (1975). *At a journal workshop.* New York: Dialogue House Library.

Robinson, J., Saberton, S., and Griffin, V. (1988). *Learning partnerships.* Toronto: OISE Press.

Rosenthal, R., and Jacobson, L. (1968). *Pygmalion in the classroom.* New York: Holt, Rinehart and Winston.

Sarason, S. B. (1966). *Psychology in community setting.* New York: Wiley.

Sarason, S. B. (1972). *The creation of settings and future societies.* San Francisco: Jossey-Bass.

Sarason, S. B. (1984). *The culture of the school and the problem of change.* Boston: Allyn Bacon.

Sarason, S. B. (1990a). *The predictable failure of educational reform.* San Francisco: Jossey-Bass.

Sarason, S. B. (1990b). *The challenge of art to psychology.* New Haven: Yale University Press.

Schein, E. H. (1990). Organizational cultures. *American Psychologist, 45,* 109-119.

Schon, D. (1983). *The reflective practitioner.* New York: Basic Books.

Schon, D. (1987). *Educating the reflective practitioner.* San Francisco: Jossey-Bass.

Sumarah, J. (1985). *The therapy of L'Arche: A model of shared living.* Unpublished doctoral dissertation. University of Toronto (OISE).

Van Cauwerberghe, V. (1988). *A search for a model to effect change through an inservice process.* Unpublished doctoral dissertation. University of Toronto (OISE).

Warren, M. Q. (1966). Interpersonal maturity level classification, Juvenile. Sacramento, CA: California Youth Authority.

Waterman, R. H. (1987). *The renewal factor.* New York: Bantam.

Yabroff, W. (1990). *The inner image.* Palo Alto: Counselling Psychology Press.

INDEX

About the Author

David Hunt is currently a Professor of Applied Psychology at the Ontario Institute for Studies in Education. In 1984, he received the Whitworth Award from the Canadian Educational Association for a distinguished contribution to educational research. In 1986, he received an Honorary Doctorate of Philosophy from the University of Helsinki. In 1989 he received the Award for Outstanding Contribution to University Teaching presented by the Ontario Council for University Faculty Associations. David Hunt has written several books and numerous articles in psychology and education.